DIABETES

DIABETES

A new & complete guide to healthier living for parents, children & young adults with insulin-dependent diabetes

by LEE DUCAT
& SHERRY SUIB COHEN

PERENNIAL LIBRARY

Harper & Row, Publishers, New York
Grand Rapids, Philadelphia, St. Louis, San Francisco
London, Singapore, Sydney, Tokyo, Toronto

To our children:
Larry, Marjorie, Allan, Jennifer, and Adam
May *their* children be born free of illness

And to the children,
the young adults, and the parents of JDF
without whom this book could not have been written

A hardcover edition of this work is published by Harper & Row,
Publishers, Inc.

First PERENNIAL LIBRARY edition published 1985.

Library of Congress Cataloging in Publication Data

Ducat, Lee.
    Diabetes, a new and complete guide to healthier
living for parents, children, and young adults with
insulin-dependent diabetes.

    Includes index.
    1. Diabetes in children.   2. Diabetes—Care and
hygiene.   I. Cohen, Sherry Suib.   II. Title.
RJ420.D5D83   1983   618.92'462   82-48661
ISBN 0-06-015153-6
ISBN 0-06-091281-2 (pbk.)

90   RRD   10   9   8   7   6   5   4   3

CONTENTS

ACKNOWLEDGMENTS

There were so many who helped. Thanks to:

The hundreds of men, women, and children of JDF who told the truth to us and to each other about what works and what doesn't work

The impassioned doctors and scientists who spent hours exploring insulin-dependent diabetes with us

Lawrence P. Ashmead, an editor in the finest tradition of book people

Senator Richard S. Schweiker, whose efforts made diabetes research a reality

Dina Merrill, the angel who provided elegance and inspiration

Dr. Robert Kaye, whose vision was behind the birth of JDF

Dr. Paul Lacy, whose friendship sustains us and whose brilliance is our finest hope for a cure

Dr. Arthur Rubenstein, a constant and respected adviser

Dr. Jørn Nerup, who took us to Europe and shared his wisdom

Dr. Henry Dolger, a trusted friend and mentor

Dr. Oscar Crofford, who steered a steady course for the diabetes commission

Bibs Orr, Lee's sister, who has always been there for her

Ed Ducat, who provided money and emotional support to start and build JDF

Carol Lurie, alter ego and adviser, without whom none of it would be possible

Connie Clausen, who brought Sherry and Lee together for this book

Joan Ratner Heilman, a very generous colleague

B. J. DeAngeles, Oliver Picher, and Anne Melanson, who organized meetings, typed, and proofed with verve and dedication

INTRODUCTION
by Paul Lacy, M.D.

This is a book which could not have been written a decade ago. In the early seventies the public still refused to acknowledge the existence of diabetes in themselves or in their family; the medical community still assumed that they alone were responsible for the treatment of the diabetic; our government was still providing a mere pittance of funds for research in diabetes; Lee Ducat, mother of a diabetic child, had just decided to abandon one career and devote her life to changing these three so-called givens of the early seventies. These three precepts have changed primarily due to the dedicated efforts of this remarkable woman. In bringing about these changes she founded the Juvenile Diabetes Foundation, served on the National Diabetes Commission, attended scientific conferences on diabetes, and talked with innumerable parents, diabetics, physicians, scientists and congressmen about diabetes. This wealth of knowledge and experience provided the background for writing this guide to healthier living for the parents, children and young adults with insulin-dependent diabetes.

The book provides helpful, practical suggestions for meeting the challenges of dealing with diabetes when the individual is under five years of age, between five and twelve, an adolescent, or an adult. Questions ranging from "What do I do on Halloween?" to "Should I tell my date I have diabetes?" to "Should I marry a diabetic?" are discussed openly with suggestions and experiences of others to assist in providing answers.

Another theme of the book is to stimulate self-advocacy in diabetics and their families in order to assure that they obtain the knowledge necessary for them to assume their responsible role in the treatment program and that proper care is being provided for them. These are questions and attitudes that have been ignored in the past and yet are of vital importance to their physical and mental health. The book is written with a spirit of optimism, with moments of humor and pathos, and with the underlying precept that knowledge will free you from fear. I believe this book will be of great value to diabetics, their parents, their brothers and sisters, their grandparents, their aunts and uncles, their friends, and their physicians in serving as a practical guide to healthier living with diabetes.

TO THE READER:
A Personal Note

You are holding a life-saver in your hands.

This is not a scientific treatise with detailed management techniques of the disease known as juvenile diabetes. There are many of those and, indeed, some of the best are listed in the back of this book.

What this book is is a *coping* manual, a practical guide, which includes the tips and touts about things that work and things that don't work; survival techniques for the person with insulin-dependent diabetes that few doctors and no authors thought you needed—until now. You won't find specific calorie guides here or "ideal height and weight guides"; those you can find in a hundred other places should you be interested. The information in these pages has been culled from the experiences of patients, families, and doctors involved in the Juvenile Diabetes Foundation (JDF), founded in 1970 by Lee Ducat. They were eager to help and share. If you can find even *one* suggestion that will make the life of someone you love who has insulin-dependent diabetes more comfortable, it will be worth the price of the book. But you will find many suggestions. We guarantee it.

Almost 2 million of the 10 million people who have diabetes have insulin-dependent diabetes, or as it used to be known, juvenile diabetes, and most of these are children and young people. That's a whole lot of young people. If they can learn to keep their diabetes under control they can probably live happy lives not very different from anyone else. We say probably, because the other thing this book is is honest. Some will not be so happy, because diabetes is an awful disease that sometimes creates complications no matter how careful people are. So there—it's out: all is not merry sunshine, even if many doctors and authors would have you think it.

But the good news is that we live in a time when diabetes management is revolutionized; when promise of the good life, and even cure, is making the atmosphere heavy with excitement for those involved in research and medicine and everyday coping. Today, people with insulin-dependent diabetes can reasonably expect to indulge in sports, marry, have healthy children and a fairly normal life span. And since progress is in the air, the goal is to keep the diabetic baby, child, adolescent, and young adult as healthy as possible, as complication-free as possible, as emotionally *whole* as possible so that he can reap the full advantages of the cure that has to come. There is hope and optimism. But first we have to get through today. And tomorrow.

Although this book has been a totally joint effort between Lee's extraordinary expertise and contacts in the field of insulin-dependent diabetes and Sherry's writing, research and interviewing skills, the first person singular "I" in the text is Lee. A word about gender usage: the old way was to refer to everyone as "he." The new way seems to be just as inaccurate because it says, "We know there are 'shes' out there, but for ease of language, forgive us if we still only say 'he.'"

These writers, both being female, refuse the old *and* the new gender applications. In this book, therefore, the reader will find references to both "he" and "she." It seems only fair.

PRELUDE

by Lee Ducat

Certain moments of my life refuse to be forgotten. They cling stubbornly to the corners of my mind, perfectly preserved vignettes that, whether I will them to or not, play over and over in almost microscopic detail. Of all these moments, there is one that brings a shudder even now.... The clock on the wall, its hands pushing toward the hour of three. The sound of a key setting the tumblers of the front door lock into motion, followed by the sudden intrusion of February's chill air. That frozen look in Edwin's eyes—the eyes of a man trying hard, perhaps too hard, to control some terrible hurt—and the pressure of his fingers digging into my arms. Then the words, so awkwardly spoken between husband and wife:

"Lee, the blood tests have come in. Our son has diabetes."

Years before, when Edwin and I were students at the University of Pennsylvania, we seemed to think of little else but one day getting married, having a brood of beautiful and healthy babies, grabbing for ourselves and our family a piece of the good life, *à la* postwar America. After graduation, we chased our dream to a tiny middle-class neighborhood of look-alike rowhouses tucked away along Philadelphia's northern limits—a block that boasted more youngsters per square inch than probably any other in the city. In short order, we dutifully contributed three little ones to the melee: Larry, Marjorie, and Allan. Every morning, along with all the other men on Lankenau Road, Edwin trooped off to work, to make his name (dared we hope for a fortune as well?) by the hospitals he built. And I, as did all the other women, stayed behind to cook the meals, clean the house, and, generally, hone my maternal skills. Carbon copies, we were—obdurate believers in white picket fences, pink-cheeked children, pie-in-the-sky executive suites, and happily-ever-afters.

With the winter of 1965, however, the lives of the five Ducats became very different from those around us. It began with a vague complaint, "Mommy, I don't feel good." Larry was nine years old at the time, a wonderfully rambunctious, tow-headed kid with sparkling brown eyes, an already well-defined streak of independence, and a maniacal devotion to Little League. Not too small, not too short, he seemed almost rudely healthy, blessed with a store of energy that I, thirty-two and trudging inexorably toward middle age, couldn't help but covet. Yet, looking down at him that evening, I suddenly saw a pale little boy, tugging at my elbow and whining in a very babyish way that he had no strength. Just three months before, he had gone through a bout of influenza, and although the symptoms weren't quite the same, I figured we were in for an encore. I calmly sent him packing into bed, gave him some aspirins, plied him with liquids and, as I turned out the light, sighed to myself, "This, too, shall pass."

But by the next day, it hadn't. Still wan and listless, still whimpering that he felt weak, he had developed an insatiable thirst, and his trips to the bathroom were increasing proportionately; his temperature, oddly enough, had slipped below normal to 97.1 degrees. I was concerned but not alarmed—at least not until later that afternoon when a gang of Larry's friends knocked at the door and asked if he could come outside to play. Knowing that he'd want to, regardless of how badly he was faring, I braced myself for a battle royal. Instead, I heard him say, "No, Mom, tell 'em I can't." And with that, I immediately picked up the telephone and made an appointment with his pediatrician for the following morning.

Larry got what appeared to me to be a complete physical examination. The doctor looked in his eyes and his ears, up his nose, down his throat, and then, smiling, delivered his pronouncement. "Doesn't look like anything to me," he assured. "If I were you, I'd send Larry right back to school." He gave me a wink, as if to say, "This kid's perfectly okay, lady. He's playing hookey." As I piled my son back into the car, I felt a grand rush of relief, as well as a slight blush of embarrassment for having momentarily succumbed to parental hysteria. As for Larry . . . well, I didn't need a medical degree to cure his school-itis.

We hadn't driven more than a few blocks, though, before an incredible thought flashed into my head. It hit like a sledgehammer tossed from somewhere on high. What am I doing? This child is definitely not okay. I'm his mother, and I know something is wrong. Very wrong. Once home, I literally hauled Larry up the stairs to the bathroom and set him down on the scale. To my horror, I discovered he had lost five pounds—proof enough for me that the doctor was mistaken, that Larry was indeed a desperately sick boy. The nearest hospital was only a five-minute ride away; we were there in three. By a quirk of fate, my husband had helped to build it and in the process had come to know the staff physicians, including the one in charge of the laboratory. Maybe for that reason he consented so quickly to perform a battery of blood tests. Or perhaps I simply scared him into it, standing in his office like some madwoman, clutching a forlornly white-faced kid. Whatever his motivation, he took the blood samples and promised us the results by the next day.

Over the twenty-four hours that followed, Larry dropped another two pounds and continued to urinate with frightening frequency. The symptoms were growing stronger, but for the life of me, I did not know what they meant. In the past, when any of the children had been ill, I invariably found comfort in the idea that, whatever the malady, it was temporary; they would rebound. But this was somehow different, and for once, an unsettling feeling of permanency nagged at me. In my mind, I began assembling a list of diseases—one more debilitating than the other—and was still torturing myself with it when my husband arrived home that afternoon with the diagnosis.

"Our son has diabetes," he said.

Impossible. Diabetes was an affliction of old age, of doddering great aunts and plump grandparents; it was the price one paid for a lifetime of overindulgence in cake and candies. Diabetes didn't happen to a child of nine, a child of mine. But . . . dammit . . . it had. Suddenly, it was as if all the curtains had been drawn in our lively little rowhouse, as if all the noises of the world sounded at once in bewildering cacophony. At the center of my brain, like a neon sign, two words began flashing: "It's incurable. It's incurable. It's incurable." And I fainted.

Edwin lifted me to my feet and held me there—held me tightly as though he thought that, by some process of osmosis, he could fill me with his strength. "You've got to pull yourself together," he instructed, his voice both demanding and pleading. "You've got to do it for Larry." He was right, of course. At that moment, our son was lying upstairs, sicker than either of us had imagined and becoming more so by the minute. Quickly making arrangements for the care of our two younger children, we packed Larry's suitcase with pajamas and a robe, scooped him out of his bed, and took off for the hospital.

To say that the doctors there were supportive would be classic understatement. Throughout the week of Larry's initial confinement, they rallied around us with outstretched arms and words of good cheer. They had been able to stabilize Larry's condition rather rapidly, they informed us; the prognosis was excellent; he would be returning home shortly. "Lee, you should thank God your son only has diabetes," one of them counseled, with a confidence intended to be infectious. "He can live with it and probably be more healthy than anyone else because he will take better care of himself. He's a very lucky little boy."

I suppose, deep inside, I was not convinced that Larry was lucky at all, or that he'd be a perfectly normal child and, one day, a perfectly normal adult. My intellect told me that this youngster, who would have to depend on insulin and the extraordinary use of syringes and needles every day for the rest of his life, was not fortunate. An illness that could not be cured remained, to my way of thinking, an illness forever. Yet, as a parent hungry for even the smallest shred of hope, I wanted desperately to believe ... to believe that insulin-dependent diabetes was, as the physicians so reassuringly described it, an "okay disease."

And that's how it all started—with Larry and Edwin and me being fed the Big Lie—a benign Big Lie that was kindly meant to salve our fears, but a lie nevertheless. Because diabetes is not an "okay" disease. And a diabetic child is only a "very lucky little boy" if you're measuring diabetes against something that's going to kill, maim, or distort you in the near future.

We *were* lucky to find friends and doctors who would help us through the myriad everyday decisions on how to live with diabetes and how best to manage Larry's health and his and our psychological well-being. It was never easy, though, and never, never possible to ignore, for even one day, this "okay" disease.

The myth continues to this very moment. Most people still think of the diabetic as the kid who has to take these shots (granted they're a nuisance), can't eat hot fudge sundaes, but who otherwise is home free, without a worry in the world. Insulin cures diabetes, doesn't it? Well, no, it doesn't. Nothing cures it ... yet.

But a whole lot of things and people make it livable with.

If you or someone you love is one of the 2 million people in this nation under thirty with insulin-dependent diabetes, you know that it's a way of life, demanding constant physical and psychological adjustments. You know that from the moment of diagnosis, so much that was sure became unsure; so much of the daily living became a question. And without the answers to at least some of those questions, life can really be sheer hell.

Thus this book. I've read too much Pollyanna preaching, heard too many lies to be satisfied with anything but truth. And truth comes from doctors and other experts, yes; but most of all, the important truths come from the parents who live with the disease and the people who have the disease. They know best what works and what doesn't, what's hype and what isn't. They are the ordinary people who directly and indirectly have had the extraordinary experience of diabetes. It's to them, along with the experts, that I've gone for this book.

I wish someone had written such a book for me when Larry was first diagnosed. I had so many problems, so many scared moments, so many everyday decisions to make that couldn't be helped by the polemic generalizations of most books. I needed a how-to book, a help book. A primer, if you will.

Here it is, then. A primer of coping. We have come together to share the wealth of practical knowledge we've accumulated.

Diabetes research accelerates, in no small part because of the Juvenile Diabetes Foundation. Already we've learned how to create longer, healthier, easier lives for insulin-dependent diabetics. And if a true cure is still a pie-in-the-sky dream, there are finally ways to live a meat and potatoes, good, wholesome and hearty life, even if you have diabetes. One day, I guarantee it, I'll stake my life on it, you'll be able to *eat* that pie-in-the-sky—with a double scoop of ice cream on top.

The purpose of this book is to make you aware of the progress of diabetes and provide information about the disease. The assessment of symptoms requires an expert. Proper diagnosis and therapy of all symptoms connected with diabetes, real or apparent, call for careful attention to your complaints by your doctor.

1 SUGAR BABIES

They were the parents of the littlest diabetics, the sugar babies, and they came into the large meeting room, two by two and sometimes one by one, very much alone. They came out on an awesomely snowy night to find answers because they were very new at this business of heartbreak and worry and they instinctively felt that in numbers, there was information and solace. They were actually that throwback to the seventies, an honest-to-goodness encounter group, and in encountering each other, they found not only answers but strengths, solutions, and even a laugh or two. Make no mistake; none was there for charitable reasons. Each hoped that by probing the common soreness, not only blame but a true healing could be discovered. It was.

Although the average age of juvenile diabetes onset in children is from ten to eleven years, the disease has appeared as early as eleven days of life, and 4 to 5 percent of the total number of children with diabetes get it when they're under two. The babies in this encounter group of parents ranged in age from two months to four years, with the exception of a thirteen-year-old whose parents were invited to show the others that diabetic babies and their parents really can survive each other's ineptitudes and traumas. And almost all of the parents that cold white night had a similar tale of discovery.

Brenda:

Beth was fourteen months old and I'd been noticing that her diapers were really drenched every time I looked—I mean soaked up to here . . . the sheets, the pad, the whole crib was *floating.* She'd developed a bad diaper rash, it wasn't healing, and she'd been pretty drowsy for days. Also, I noticed she was constantly asking me for water.

"It's good for her to drink a lot," my pediatrician assured me. "Look how hot it is out—she'll be just fine."

I wasn't so sure. I noticed that she'd lost a little over a pound in a week and a half and there weren't too many pounds *to* her.

"Don't be silly—she's losing her baby fat," said my sister.

I wondered why she was losing her baby fat when she was still a baby.

The doctor prescribed antibiotics for the rash, which he diagnosed as a staph infection, and red meat for her lethargy. Neither worked, and Beth was getting thirstier by the moment. The turning point came on Sunday afternoon when she'd asked for her fourth glass of water in a half hour and when I didn't get it fast enough, she crawled, with obvious desperation, to my coffee table, pulled down a small vase with daffodils, and began drinking the flower water.

"Oh, God," I said to my husband. "Something's terribly wrong."

And so the parents shared the way they found out that diabetes was to be a part of their lives. A thirsty, cranky baby with drenched diapers; a little girl acting funny, having temper tantrums for no reason at all; a mother with a close-to-coma baby in her arms being asked to fill out insurance information at the hospital; a little boy refusing to get out of a urine-soaked bed on Christmas Day even though he knew all his presents were waiting. . . .

From the encounter group that evening came more than stories. What emerged was parent-to-parent hard information and tips, things to watch out for, things to get, things to think about, the newest devices, the newest research, the best doctors. And so we held other encounter groups with parents of nursery-school-aged children and parents of adolescents and parents of young adults. The information gleaned was astounding—much better than listening to hundreds of learned doctors who don't live with the problems and successes. Then we met with the kids: local chapters of the Juvenile Diabetes Foundation (JDF) all over the country set up meetings with their junior members. And *that* was an education.

That's why we wrote this book. To share all the good stuff with you.

First of all, you ought to know that it is rare for a child to be born with diabetes and rarer still for that child to survive infancy. If the baby is especially sturdy, he has a chance—but only if the attending physician immediately administers blood sugar tests and begins a regimen of minute amounts of insulin. Which doesn't often happen. Usually, what does happen is that the newborn will deteriorate at such a rapid clip that, by the time diabetes is suspected, it's too late to avert tragedy. But it's a different story if diabetes comes between infancy and the age of five. You have a fighting chance and more than a fighting chance that your baby will not only survive but live to lead a productive and relatively healthy life. And so, you're in that position now. Your physician has, by a variety of methods, diagnosed your up-till-now healthy baby as having diabetes mellitus—insulin-requiring diabetes. What happens next?

SUGAR BABIES AT THE HOSPITAL

Okay, so your baby has been tentatively diagnosed as diabetic. Numb, frightened, you're almost relieved when the doctor tells you that the best thing for the whole family is to hospitalize the baby for a week or so. The baby's not *that* sick and you really don't know why he requires hospitalization. But secretly you're happy that the whole thing is temporarily out of your hands. It's the hospital's job, now. Right? Wrong.

Unlike the usual hospital stay, where the parents' only responsibility is to provide tender loving care for their children, during this hospitalization you have a real job to do. The family's eight- to ten-day hospital experience will lay the foundation for the entire future management of your child's illness. If all goes well, it will provide the tools, techniques, and psychological attitudes that will carry you smoothly through the years. You'll learn many things during this time, but the most important thing you can learn is that this is the beginning of the education that will make you far more capable than even your doctor in managing your child's diabetes. Because every case is different and everyone responds individually to treatments and regimens, you will eventually come to respect your own judgments and the patient's body rhythms more than anything else. If you have to get diabetes, this is the most helpful time to do it. Important new advances are with us already and there's much exciting news about possibilities hovering right around the corner.

For the first time in history, today a diabetic can choose his own treatments, in consultation with the best doctors he can find, because there are alternative treatments from which to choose. Which is why this first hospital experience (with any luck, it will be the last one, also) is very important: it *should* give you an overview of what's available and what's possible.

Naturally, the care and attention you'll receive will depend on the size, character, and relative wealth of the medical institution; still, any good hospital will provide certain essentials in instruction, treatment, and modern equipment, and you should not settle for less. The following is presented as an outside guide to the care and instruction you can reasonably expect in a good hospital.

If you suspect that your child's treatment is not what it should be, turn into a mother-monster, a father-fighter—anything that will make you a *parent advocate.* You'll read that term quite a bit in this book. It means only that you are the best possible person to stick up for your kid. Even if you've been a shrinking violet all your life and have never questioned authority, now is the time to reconstitute your personality. If you think your little one is being shortchanged by carelessness, callousness, or incompetence, ask questions, request necessary changes, *insist* upon humane, quality attention!

WHAT SHOULD HAPPEN AT THE HOSPITAL

Many things should happen and most of them come under the heading of five categories suggested by Dr. Lester Baker, Professor of Pediatrics at the University of Pennsylvania School of Medicine and director of the Division of Endocrinology/Diabetes at the Children's Hospital in Philadelphia:

A Specific Diagnosis

This is the easy part. It's not difficult to diagnose diabetes with the easy availability of blood and urine tests and the recognition of the three "polys"—*polyuria,* excessive urination; *polydipsia,* an awesome thirst, which cannot be satisfied; and *polyhagia,* the least common of the symptoms, which involves enormous hunger.

Symptoms: Your toddler may have been dragging around for days because of a heaviness in his legs, dizziness, or general lethargy. Your infant might have been unaccountably cranky. If the condition was unnoticed for too long, your child might have been brought to the hospital in a state of keto-acidosis (a condition that arises when toxic acids accumulate in the bloodstream, ketones appear in the urine, and the patient becomes dehydrated) or in a diabetic coma.

If it's not difficult to diagnose diabetes, how come your pediatrician didn't call it when he first saw your child? As easy as it is to diagnose, that's how easy it is to miss, because the symptoms can often be confused with those of urinary infections, anemia, behavioral problems, and other diseases. In fact, diagnosis of diabetes is either not made or delayed in 50 percent of children on their first visits to their doctors. Particularly difficult to diagnose are very small patients with very small or nonexistent vocabularies. Brain-damaged children often fail to recognize their own thirst and so present one less important symptom to their doctors. However, there is a growing public awareness of diabetes symptoms and many concerned parents are actually pushing their doctors into making urine tests when there are questions. A positive test of urine for glucose is a clear-cut diagnosis.

Make Him Feel Better

After the diagnosis, the next order of business in the hospital is to restore your child's sense of health and well-being as soon as possible. This can be accomplished soon—in a day or so, at most—in all but the most seriously ill children. If a child is very sick when he is admitted, in diabetic keto-acidosis or in coma, he will be treated immediately with insulin, medication, and fluids administered intravenously. The doctor will be concerned with all of the things that may be life-threatening, such as cardiovascular collapse, shock, and the profound acidosis itself. Blood glucose concentrations *should* be taken hourly, at this point, says Dr. Lester Baker, to assess the efficacy of treatment. Your child should be closely watched by medical personnel to monitor his state of consciousness, blood pressure, and fluid input-output. If these things are not happening, get the senior person in charge to do something about it. This is a wonderful time to start becoming an effective parent advocate. On the other hand, if you truly sense that the medical personnel are alert and sensitive to your child's illness, don't be a nag. Allow them to do their job, question whatever you don't understand, and be there for your child, touching him lovingly, as much as possible.

If your newly diagnosed diabetic child has milder symptoms, he will probably be treated with low doses of insulin injections that will make him feel better, wonderfully soon. Experts agree that it's desirable to spend a lot of loving, supportive time with a hospitalized small child, even sleeping in his room if that is feasible. Many parents take turns staying the night. Most hospitals, sometimes grudgingly but who cares, will permit this relaxation of rules if the parent firmly requests it. (Niceness doesn't hurt either.)

Me—An Artificial Pancreas?

Yes. Until your baby is old enough to do the job himself, you've got to learn to be a substitute for his pancreas ... which means that the hospital should provide a thorough educational program teaching you to do just that. Not only do you have to learn how and when to provide the insulin that most normally functioning pancreases do automatically, you also must learn how to make judgments and decisions that will help you solve the daily problems that arise. You will, in fact, says Dr. Baker, "become your child's primary physician while the physician acts as consultant."

All that takes work and concentration, and no one expects you to grasp the masses of information you'll be bombarded with the first time, or even the second time it's presented. You are no doubt feeling dizzy with shock and worry, but try to listen carefully and ask many questions anyway. Don't be afraid they'll think you're dumb/neurotic/overprotective/over-reactive/childish ... anything! It's hard to think straight when you've been hit with a brick, and everyone knows it.

The program itself: don't accept an educational process that consists of an I TALK, YOU LISTEN attitude from the doctor. And don't accept a program of rules to memorize as if they were inscribed in stone. It's not enough.

What should happen are many conversations between you and the doctors, nutritionists, psychologists, and other members of the hospital team, which will slowly clue you into the niceties of

1. The functions of insulin and your child's particular needs.

2. Home glucose monitoring by blood or urine. Most up-to-date specialists recommend blood testing as the most effective way to obtain blood sugar control.

3. The injections: how, when, and why they're given.

4. The diabetic emergency situations: what they are, when to look for them, what to do.

An excellent book to guide you through these discussions and one to which you will constantly refer is Luther B. Travis's *An Instructional Aid on Juvenile Diabetes Mellitus* (obtainable from the South Texas Affiliate of the American Diabetes Association, P.O. Box 12946, Austin, TX 78711). It's a good idea to go over the text with your doctor, asking as many questions as come up.

The hospital educational program should also include a visit from a nutritionist who will help your family assess its eating patterns to best manage the diabetic child's diet. You'll probably end up being the healthiest family in town because a diabetic's diet is sound and healthy for all. And don't be nervous. Diet doesn't mean deprivation: a diabetic diet can be as varied and exotic as your lifestyle dictates, with a little imagination.

Psychological Support Is Not a Crutch, It's a Pillar

The hospitalization of your child during his first bout with diabetes should include some counseling for the whole family. And make no mistake, this *is* a family problem that should not ever be just the mother's responsibility. It's a time to get siblings, even grandparents, involved in the talks with the hospital psychological professionals that will help you all to air your worst fears and highest hopes. Especially wonderful at this time is the support system that other parents of diabetic children willingly provide. Your doctor should put you in touch with your local Juvenile Diabetes Foundation chapter, which can give you the names of such parents.

Even though that first phone call might be difficult, do it! Talking to parents who have been there paves the way as nothing else can.

Goal Planning

Finally, what should happen at the hospital is a discussion between you and your doctor outlining the basic goals for your child, to be colored in and implemented, of course, as the child grows. Meaningful goals should be set for each age group—preschool, middle (five to twelve years), adolescent, and young adult. The baby diabetic's parents, according to the experts at Children's Hospital in Philadelphia, should have the following goals in mind:

—avoidance of extremes of hypoglycemia (low blood sugar) and hyperglycemia (high blood sugar)

- *Hypoglycemia* leads to an insulin reaction, which is a condition that arises as blood sugar is lowered below normal levels of between 90 and 120 and too much injected insulin is circulating in the blood. This, in turn, leads to symptoms of clamminess, dizziness, shakiness. If not treated with sugar, the reaction may progress to convulsions, unconsciousness and ultimately to death.

- *Hyperglycemia*, a condition where blood sugars continue to rise because the insulin level is insufficient, is expressed by excessive thirst, urination, and nausea. This can, if not treated by insulin, lead to coma and death.

—correction of metabolic problems that may occur during common childhood illnesses so as to avoid hospitalization

—maintenance not only of physical and emotional growth for the diabetic child but of the emotional growth and health of the whole family

And that's what should *happen at that first hospitalization...*

WHAT SHOULD NOT HAPPEN AT THE HOSPITAL

There's no way to put this information into categories. The best method of setting a feeling of what is *poor* hospital practice is to read through the list that follows. Hospitals are busy places; poor hospital practices are usually the result of harried medical personnel and inadequate funding. No one means to be careless or callous. Still, understanding this does not preclude your taking an active role in trying to do something about care that may be physically or emotionally harmful to your child. Even though he's not a graduate of medical school, a parent advocate should take on some of the responsibility of his child's medical care. That is not being unreasonable or unrealistic. Let them call you a pushy parent or even a nuisance. You probably won't win any popularity contests by being a parent advocate. But the firmest, most alert-to-problems, most vocal parent almost always gets the best attention for his child.

1. Kids First, Forms Later   Let no one boondoggle you into filling out forms before care is given to a seriously ill child brought into a hospital. Too many parents have told horror stories of sitting in admittance rooms, wading through red tape, while holding a close-to-comatose child in their arms. Loudly demand to see a supervisor immediately if anyone gives you "those are the rules" garbage. Say the words "lawyer" and "malpractice suit" a lot. The best solution, of course, is for one parent to give all the necessary information while the other stays with the child to ensure that care is immediately forthcoming. If there is only one of you, the paperwork *must* wait.

2. Glucose Tolerance Testing? Not Necessary   A glucose tolerance test is a time-consuming, complicated method of diagnosing diabetes, and many doctors routinely perform this test on a sick child, suspected diabetic, when that child is brought into a hospital. Current thinking today says that the test may result in undue delay of diagnosis with further deterioration taking place in a child who should be treated, not tested, immediately. Dr. Lester Baker says that "glucose tolerance testing is usually a waste of precious time with virtually no place at all. When a doctor with a glucose finding in a urine test arranges for a glucose tolerance test, it's very possible his patient may slip, while waiting for the test to be performed, into more serious problems. A child who has a fasting blood sugar of 150 or a random after meals specimen of 180 or so has no need for the test. *Perhaps*, if you get some grays on numbers like a fasting blood sugar of 110 or an after meals sugar of 140—perhaps, then, the test might be useful. But otherwise, there can be danger in delaying treatment."

3. You're Allowed to Say: "No More!"   Often medication, fluids or nourishment need to be continuously administered through a vein (intravenously) or blood samples are required, but too often inexperienced technicians or externs who are just learning are sent to do the job. If your child's tiny arms or heels have been pricked just too many times in an attempt to find a vein or to get blood (more than three times without success we'd say is too many times), politely stop the ineffectual pricking and ask the nursing supervisor to provide someone more talented. There's no reason for your child to suffer *too much* inexperience, even when you understand that a teaching hospital's the place where people expect to learn to be expert. And anyone who walks out of your baby's room forgetting to remove a tourniquet should not be allowed back into that room—ever again.

4. Time Is of the Essence   A blood sugar test indicates what your child's blood is like at the time of testing—not four hours later. To take a blood test at eight o'clock in the morning and have the results of the test return at eleven is meaningless if you're waiting to find out what your child should eat for breakfast in order to keep his blood sugar in control. To diagnose and prescribe properly, up-to-date medical facilities ought to arrange to have blood test results within from two to three minutes to, at most, an hour. Glucose analyzers such as Chemstrips, Dextrometers, or Glucometer Reflectance Meters ought to be in close proximity to any diabetic patient. If you are in a hospital where it takes more than an hour to get blood test results, you can offer to ferry the blood samples personally down to the laboratory, wait for the results, and trot them back to the doctor. You'll probably shame them into a faster trot.

5. Pain Is Not Part of the Game   Inordinate pain from needle pricking doesn't have to be. The initial shock of a hospitalization is often such a trauma to toddlers or infants that constantly being stuck with sharp needles is just too much extra to take. If your child is particularly fearful, ask your doctor about an in-dwelling heparin lock system which, once in place, allows frequent blood to be drawn without further pricks. If that is not practicable, ask the doctor about the Autolet system marketed by Bio-Dynamics, Inc., and the Ames Company.* It's a spring-driven lancet holder that when used properly reduces the pricking pain almost totally. Jabbing a young child with only a lancet, over and over and over, compounds everyone's misery.

6. Nurses Can Panic, Too   If you see someone about to do a dumb thing, don't let a white uniform or a stethoscope intimidate you into stopping the act. One parent tells how her baby went into insulin shock and the nurse, remembering that sugar had to be supplied, grabbed the first sugar product at hand and poured it into the infant's mouth. It was powdered strawberry gelatin and naturally the baby almost choked to death as she inhaled the pink dust. Incidentally, now is not too soon to begin carrying around a tube of sugary cake gel, or Mono Gel, which is obtainable at a drugstore, or even honey (in a small vial), either of which can be safely sqeezed into a baby's mouth to provide the necessary sugar during an insulin reaction . . . whenever it might come.

* Addresses are listed under Professional Organizations and Manufacturers in the resource section at the end of this book.

7. *Just Because It Came from the Hospital Doesn't Mean It's Sacred* Question anything that sounds fluky no matter who prescribes it. We've heard of a child who absolutely refused to follow the meal plan provided for her from the hospital. The printed diet specified the same meals every day, every week of every year. After three months of eating the same food every day, the child exploded in fury. Naturally. We've also heard of a father who refused to let an intern change the insulin prescription the family's diabetologist recommended. He was right—and the intern wrong—but it took guts to stand up to an officious doctor who insisted that he was in charge of the floor rather than the specialist.

Okay, you're home from the hospital. What next?

YOUR CHILD'S DOCTOR

During the days of your child's initial hospitalization, you may have found yourself being run ragged, mentally as well as physically. Oh, to be a computer at times like these—able to accept every piece of data, organize it, store it, and call it up when needed. And, now, you have to make a crucial decision before you go home. What doctor will treat your child from this moment on? Naturally, you want the best; but how do you find it? The best is a pediatric diabetes specialist and endocrinologist with sterling qualifications, a reputation for keeping up with the latest trends in treatment, a willingness to be there when you need him, and connections with a respected hospital. That dream doctor may just be the hospital physician who stabilized your child. Or he may not be. What about your own pediatrician, the guy who got Johnny through measles, croup, and assorted other childhood traumas so far?

Your pediatrician might be absolutely top notch, but let's face it: if recognizing and treating diabetes is only a fragment of that doctor's everyday practice (and even though diabetes is far from rare, this is often the case), you can't reasonably expect him to be absolutely current with the very latest in theory and practice. So it's a good idea to have two doctors for your baby: one who will treat the whole child and not just the diabetes; and a diabetologist who is willing to work hand in hand (or phone to phone) with the regular doctor. It's been the experience of most families that this specialist often becomes a focal point in the child's later life, and often acts as an intermediary in adolescence when many teenagers resent and rebel against parental direction. At least one of these doctors, if you have two, should be available at any hour of the day or night for a phone consultation should an emergency arise—and don't hesitate to ask whether this service will be forthcoming before you decide on a doctor.

If you decide to consult with a diabetes specialist, you can best locate a good one by making inquiries at a large teaching hospital (preferably a children's hospital) in your community. Your pediatrician can also recommend such a specialist, and your local chapter of the Juvenile Diabetes Foundation is available to suggest possibilities. Another resource for suggestions is the Joslin Clinic in Boston, Massachusetts, the oldest and best-known diabetes center in the country. Or, you can consult with families of diabetics who are managing well with the doctors they've chosen. At the back of this book is a list of doctors recommended by parent members of the Juvenile Diabetes Foundation as another source for you to consider.

In any case, that decision should not be allowed to fall into the lap of the family doctor. Don't abdicate your responsibility in this matter. Take the time to gather the information you'll need to make an informed decision. If you live in a rural area and no diabetes specialist is available, perhaps you and your local doctor can hone your mutual skills and learn together how best to handle an insulin-dependent diabetic child.

A rule of thumb: If your baby seems to be growing normally, without too many insulin reactions and without convulsions or repeated hospitalizations; if he seems happy and healthy—chances are you've made the right decision. If not, change doctors fast. That is your right and your responsibility.

The Minimal Examination

No matter who your doctor is—regular pediatrician, specialist, or a team— your baby should be examined every three months. Remember *to write down* any questions you may have on a pad kept especially for that purpose, and don't hesitate to ask every one of them at the time of your appointment. If your doctor makes you feel rushed or if you are made to feel foolish for asking for the explanations, find another doctor.

Dr. Henry Dolger, Professor Emeritus at the Mount Sinai School of Medicine in New York and Consultant for Diabetes at the Mount Sinai Hospital, suggests the following routine to be included in every minimal examination.

1. Growth Check "This takes precedence over every other criterion," says Dr. Dolger. "At each visit, the doctor should measure the child's growth and weight and compare the new figures with previous height and weight figures, as well as with averages for the normal child of his age. If a child is not growing properly, we can usually assume that something is wrong with his insulin coverage. Even when tests show that the blood sugar is well controlled, the insulin may still have to be corrected in either total dosage or time-span coverage, if the growth is not what it should be. If a child is not growing properly, there might be something wrong with his insulin. Keep in mind that insulin is a growth hormone and can suppress or elevate growth."

Dr. Alicia Schiffrin, a pediatric endocrinologist with Montreal Children's Hospital, says: "Sometimes a blood sugar may look normal but the child may still have an elevated Hemoglobin A1c Test because the blood has been tested during the day when the child is within normal range. But at night, the child may be sleeping in high sugars. So, if there's any doubt, check his blood sugars at night. And keep this in mind: perhaps your child is short because of genetic factors having nothing to do with diabetes. It's very important to see how the child was growing before the onset of diabetes. If he was growing slowly before the diabetes set in, it's reasonable to expect he'll continue to do so. If his growth velocity changed after the onset of the disease, it may well be related to the amount of insulin he's taking."

And be sure your child is treated by a specialist, says Dr. Schiffrin. Sometimes children are growing well before the onset of the disease; they develop diabetes, are treated with an initial dose of insulin by their family doctors, and the dose is not changed as they grow—because the doctors simply don't know that insulin must be adjusted constantly. These children will be very thin, says Dr. Schiffrin, and their growth will be quite poor.

2. A Mouth Examination to Check Gums   Dentists often are able to make an initial diagnosis of diabetes because unusually purplish or spongy gums reflect a condition of decalcification, frequently present with a urine blood sugar spill. The doctor knows that suspicious-looking gums can be a true indicator of poor blood sugar management.

3. An Eye Check   Because diabetics are more likely to develop a deterioration of the small blood vessels that nourish the retina—a condition known as *retinopathy*—regular eye examinations are essential. Often the pediatrician or the diabetes specialist is the first to spot problems.

Dr. Francis L'Esperance, Jr., Associate Professor of Clinical Ophthalmology at the College of Physicians and Surgeons, Columbia University, in New York, says that as a general rule every patient who has diabetes diagnosed should to go to the eye specialist immediately after diagnosis *and the specialist should be an ophthalmologist who is a retina or diabetic retinopathy expert.* If the child is an infant, it's not necessary to see the eye specialist yearly because (1) retinopathy takes about eight years to develop, and (2) it's very difficult to find a child at that age who'd be cooperative enough to be examined thoroughly. Once a child who's been diagnosed at an early age reaches four or five, even though chances are less than 1 percent that she'll have any kind of retinopathy, it's a good idea to see the ophthalmologist, and yearly thereafter.

Dr. L'Esperance cautions that diabetes may be officially diagnosed at ten years of age but it's quite possible that the child had a mild diabetes, unnoticed, even before. If this happens, eye problems could have been developing unnoticed. When the disease is finally diagnosed and the ten-year-old sees an eye specialist, he may already have a visible retinal hemorrhage. The doctor will watch this carefully, after treatment, and will continue to look for broken blood vessels in the back of the patient's eye. If retinopathy seems to be worsening, the patient may be asked to come back after a six-month hiatus, instead of yearly. If the retinopathy is very active, a visit every three months is probably desirable.

4. Glycohemoglobin Test (Otherwise Known as the Hemoglobin Alc Test)   This is a test that tells you *more* than how your child is doing today or this week with blood sugar control. It gives an accurate assessment of how effective control has been over the past three months. How does it work? Hemoglobin Alc is hemoglobin with glucose attached to it. If you have a high sugar concentration in your blood, it's reflected by the amount of glucose that is attached to the blood cells which stays there for two or three months. When your doctor gives your child this test, he will be able to make an accurate assessment of how effective control has been over the past three months. A normal level ranges between 4 and 7 percent (depending on the methods used by the laboratory); higher than that tells you that blood glucose control needs revamping.

Can the test ever be wrong? Sure, says Dr. Anthony Cerami, Professor of Medicine and Biochemistry at Rockefeller University in New York. "Accuracy depends on the person who takes the test, and the competency of the laboratory. In our laboratories we have a general rule that any clinical test that reads abnormal is done again." Don't be surprised if your child's test is slightly higher than normal. Dr. Cerami notes that very few patients are ever in perfect control, even though most medical evidence points to the theory that better control means fewer complications.

The Hemoglobin Alc Test is a wonderful tool. Not only does it give you information as to your child's blood sugar status, but it also is an invaluable help when prescribing proper amounts of insulin, diet, and food. It's an essential part of every three-month "seasonal" examination. Why do we call it seasonal? Because diabetes management changes drastically with the seasons, as Dr. Dolger points out. When daylight savings time comes around and the days lengthen, there's more physical activity involved in your baby's life—outside and inside. As the baby or toddler becomes more active, he/she will need less insulin. The advent of winter and fall means more head colds, and sick days mean insulin adjustments. Summer is also associated with stomach viruses and vomiting, as well as camp and weekend travel—all of which mean changes in care. Thus diabetes is a seasonal disease when it comes to treatment.

The honeymoon is over ... What, so fast?

After your child has been diagnosed and treatment has started, something very nice and something very cruel happens ... and it's the same thing. The nice part is that within several months, a remission of diabetes occurs in many children. They seem to get all better: their blood sugar is normal, they begin to secrete normal amounts of insulin naturally.

Suddenly, the insulin requirement gets considerably lower. And then even lower. Some children may not need any at all, after a while. Parents and doctors who are not knowledgeable are euphoric: it looks like a miraculous recovery. But the cruel thing happens soon, after only a few weeks or perhaps months. Your child may have a cold, or fall hard while he's learning to walk—any simple infection or minor trauma can precipitate what happens, which is that the diabetes returns.

The recovery was short-lived. This is called the honeymoon stage, and if you're not prepared for it, the disappointment can be enormous. The very best thing you can do is to understand that diabetes is a chronic disease. Your child will always have it, and to hope for miracles, this week, this year, is not reasonable. However, and it's a big however, you *can* hope for miracles soon. We seem to be on the crest of discovery with diabetes, and there are all sorts of possibilities just beyond the horizon—even a little closer. More of this in Chapter 5. As far as today goes, you ought to arm yourself with knowledge; and one of the things you ought to know about— even if it's a big downer—is this "honeymoon" remission business.

METHODS OF HOME GLUCOSE MONITORING

In the hospital, your baby's diabetes has been brought under control. Now, in order to keep the blood sugar stabilized, you're going to have to keep close track of what's going on inside that little body.

There are two ways to do it. You can check on sugar levels by testing either the urine or the blood.

In this chapter, you'll learn how to do both, because this whole book is about choice. Until recently, there was no choice. Diabetics were wholly dependent on urine testing. Blood monitoring was a mysterious process that only a person in a white coat understood, and even he had to send the whole shebang to a laboratory to get readings. Not so today. Modern medicine provides, at last, alternatives, and that's what humanizes people—and the management of diabetes also.

So much for the choices. Now for preferences and informed opinions.

I unequivocally recommend the blood-testing method. So do most knowledgeable doctors in the field of juvenile diabetes. For instance, Dr. Alan Rubin, who is Assistant Clinical Professor of Medicine at the University of San Francisco Medical College and director of the San Francisco Diabetes Medical Group, says: "Patients' self testing of blood sugar is the proper way to monitor treatment in diabetes mellitus and it is no longer acceptable or appropriate to advocate, perform, or teach testing of the urine in diabetes mellitus."

Pretty strong words, all right, but they're echoed today by many leaders in the field of diabetes research who believe that home blood testing is probably the most important advance in recent diabetes history. Dr. Rubin says that urine testing can be compared to "a baseball batter attempting to hit a baseball by following its shadow on the ground: depending on whether it's a shady or sunny day, his view of that shadow will change each time." Urine testing is indeed, many of us feel, so imprecise because it *cannot* do more than it can do (specific example of this appear in the pros and cons section that follows). It reflects just a shadow of what is really happening in your child's body because urine sugars don't tell you what's happening that moment; they only reflect sugars *after* they're dumped by the blood into the urine. It's possible, therefore, that someone could have a high urine sugar reading of 4+ and a low blood sugar reading of 60—and only the latter would be accurate. When testing urine, either with tapes or test tubes, it's *color* that tells you the percentage of sugar that's in your urine. A certain color will tell you that your urine has a certain percent of sugar and this is read as a range of from 0 sugar to 5+ sugar. A urine reading of 4+ would indicate a very high percentage of sugar in your urine.

There surely are arguments against home blood sugar testing, but there are good answers to every one of them. Opponents of the method say that most patients will be unwilling to stick themselves several times a day because of the inherent pain. Inventions like the Autolet, an almost pain-free pricking device, cancel out that theory. Many physicians say that the cost of the blood-testing equipment is too high. All the equipment you need is less expensive than just one day in the intensive care unit of a hospital, where many patients, misjudging their true sugar levels from shady urine tests, end up. Still other doctors say that many patients are not smart enough to deal with blood tests and that the whole thing depresses them, anyway. Tests have shown that patients from every age and socioeconomic level have been successfully taught to measure their blood sugar; and, far from depressing patients, it makes them feel optimistic that for the first time they have good control and can *do* something about their disease.

Don't misunderstand: urine testing should still be done *in addition,* on sick days, to see if there are ketones in the urine—a sign of trouble, which usually means more insulin is needed immediately (usually 2–4 units of regular or short-acting, but ask your own doctor).

So there you have it—an impassioned argument for using home blood testing instead of urine testing. Talk to your own doctor, and then *you* decide, although we feel that the day is near when home blood testing will be the only method that doctors recommend for establishing excellent control. We're lucky to live at a time when it's finally available.

Home Urine Testing

When the blood glucose level exceeds a certain threshold (about 150 to 180 mg.), sugar begins to spill over into the urine. This point is called the *renal threshold* and it differs among people and changes, sometimes, even in your own body. Little ones usually have lower than normal renal thresholds; that is, their sugar begins to spill sometimes even before it reaches that 150–180 level. An infant may thus show sugar in his urine but have a normal blood sugar.

What does the testing show? The general assumption of those who test their urine for sugar is that if sugar appears in the urine, the sugar that was circulating in the blood during the past few hours before the test was higher than normal. The first step in urine testing is to have the doctor establish your baby's renal threshhold. He does this by taking several blood sugar tests in a row and by doing a urine sugar test at the same time. Supposedly, once you know the level of sugar in your child's urine, you can use that information to decide what amounts of insulin, food, and exercise he should have for the day. We'll give you both the advantages and disadvantages of urine testing—and then you make up your mind.

Pros and cons of urine testing

PROS	CONS
It's inexpensive.	Because children have a low renal threshold, they can spill sugar into their urine when blood sugar may be just a little high or even normal. Knowing this intellectually doesn't preclude the feeling that you should *do* something about that sugar—when you really shouldn't.
It's easy and convenient.	
It doesn't require finger pricking or cause bleeding.	
	Urine testing doesn't show you what your blood sugar is at the moment of the test; what you're getting is history, not news.
	Urine testing doesn't show you low blood sugar, which is important to know because your baby could be hypoglycemic. It only records high sugar.
	Urine sugar test results can be altered by such extraneous factors as moisture, Vitamin C, medications, aspirin. Even a sticky bun remnant on your fingers when you test can change the results. Drinking a lot of water certainly can.
	People don't love squeezing out dank diapers to retrieve urine.

If you decide to go the urine-testing route (maybe your doctor can come up with more pros), this is how to do it:

Urine testing is usually done four times a day, before each meal and at bedtime. If you are instructed to test your child's *second* void, it's because many people feel that the urine that's been collecting in the bladder all night is not indicative of the blood sugar state in the morning and that the second void is more telling of the urine sugar content of the last few hours. The way you take a second void is this: you don't test the baby's diaper after her first urination; instead, you give her a drink of water and wait until the diaper is wet again. This presents obvious problems since very few babies and toddlers are able to urinate on demand, as an adult usually can. Therefore, it's often suggested by many doctors that you ignore the whole second void theory since recent studies have even suggested that accuracy is not much, if at all, improved by the second void method.

The one thing you must remember in urine testing is that you need to get an overall pattern of your baby's blood sugar levels and isolated results are not very telling of anything. If you keep close records of the results of each test, you will be able to detect, for instance, a certain rise of sugar almost every noontime, as the chart below indicates. You'd then make adjustments in diet, activity, or medication, to compensate, after consulting with your doctor. Ideal results should really show at least two or three urine tests a day without any sugar at all:

Weekly Blood-Sugar Results

	AM	Noon	PM	Bedtime
Mon	N	N	N	N
Tues	N	1%	N	N
Wed	N	½%	N	1/10%
Thurs	N	½%	N	N
Fri	N	½%	N	N
Sat	N	1%	N	N
Sun	N	½%	N	N

As the parent of a diabetic child, you must remember that there is no such thing as a *perfectly* controlled juvenile diabetic—one in which blood sugar levels are always at a normal level. As your baby grows, she/he will be a busy and creative person with diversified activities (you hope), unable to lead a totally plannable, predictable life. So it's good to learn now, while he's still a baby, not to expect his urine to be sugar-free all the time. In fact, many doctors today don't think a child should be negative all of the time.

And here are some wise words: *do not ever feel guilty* if your child spills sugar into his urine. You can be completely reliable about diet, insulin, and exercise, and still, your little one can spill, depending on a multitude of factors that may not be under your control at all. Sugar in the urine may mean, for example, that a whopper of a cold is coming on. You'd have to be pretty bananas to blame yourself for cold viruses in the air.

There are three methods you can use to test your little child's urine. The one recommended most often for insulin-dependent diabetics is the Clinitest Two-Drop Method.

Clinitest Two-Drop Method You will need a test tube and an eyedropper.

Squeeze a few drops of urine from the baby's diaper into a cup. With the dropper, collect two drops and place them into the test tube along with ten drops of water. Add a Clinitest tablet, wait, shake gently, and when the mixture stops roiling, wait another fifteen seconds before comparing the color of the specimen with the chart provided. The colors go from blue, which is negative, to orange, which is 5 percent and requires instant attention.

Diastix   These are plastic sticks with blue paper chemical-testing areas at one end. Dip the blue part into some urine, or hold it against a diaper, which gives a pretty good reading, say most parents. Wait thirty seconds, then compare to the colors on the container in which the stick came. The range is from aqua (negative) to brown (positive). These sticks are good for trips and even for inexperienced babysitters who want to get a fast reading on their charges. They of course depend on at least one parent not being color-blind.

TIP: It's probably a good idea to use disposable diapers so as not to chance contaminating test results with soap or detergent residue.

Tes-Tape   This is a convenient roll of yellow, chemically treated tape that is torn off as needed, dipped into a urine specimen, and checked. Wait one minute before checking the colors. If the strip doesn't change color at all (stays yellow), the urine is negative. It may change to gradually darkening hues of green. If it stays at ½ percent (a reading of 3+ at the end of the minute), wait another minute before comparing colors.

CAUTION: Don't test the part of the tape you've touched with your fingers because any sugar on your fingertips may cause a false positive result.

An Ingenious Extra Bonus   Tes-Tapes or Diastix can be used, says Dr. Richard Bernstein, author of *Diabetes: The Glucograf Method for Normalizing Blood Sugar,* to dunk into foods like prepared baby foods, salad dressings, anything you might feed your baby that might (you're not sure) be laden with sugar. Dr. Bernstein believes that if they register below ½ percent on the tapes, they're probably okay to eat.

A few final words on urine testing. What do you do with the results?

Here are some suggestions. The explanation below should help you to identify what is happening with your child's blood sugar; *but always check with your physician before making substantial changes in the insulin dosage.*

- If urines are all or predominantly negative . . . Keep doing what you're doing.
- If urines are all or predominantly negative, but the baby seems to be having insulin reactions in a regular pattern . . . Give him more food,

or reduce his insulin during the period *before* the occurring reaction.
- If urines are all or mostly all negative and the baby is having reactions in no pattern . . . Give him more food, or reduce the total insulin.
- If you see sugar spilling at the same time for several days . . . Give him less food, more exercise, or increase insulin before time of spill.
- If spilling occurs with no pattern at all, but insulin reactions occur when insulin is raised or food decreased . . . Check out peak actions on insulin, and check out his activity, food, and illness or stress possibilities (perhaps multiple doses of insulin will help). Check with your doctor as to raises in insulin doses.
- If you see a gradually increasing spill over three or four days . . . Try a raise in insulin or less food. Also check out any infection or stress. Growing can cause a blood sugar rise.

Testing for Ketones

Ketones are the substances that come about when fat and muscle are burned for fuel because the body's cells are not getting glucose. When ketones and 2 or more per cent of sugar are present in the urine, it spells trouble. Let the situation continue and your baby is on his way to a diabetic coma. Illnesses or infections are times when this combination is particularly possible. Sugar and ketones can also come from extraordinary stress.

It's simple to test for ketones. The Ames Company puts out Ketostix, a chemically treated paper strip. If you dip it into urine, wait fifteen seconds, and then check its color, you'll soon know if you have any. If the color does not change, there are no ketones (or acetones) present. Lavender means some ketones are present. If it turns deep purple, your baby has a large amount of ketones.

The same company also puts out Acetest tablets. If you put a drop of urine on the tablet, and wait thirty seconds, the same colors give you the whole story. Always keep a record of your results to have for your own information and to give to your doctor. You can buy a compact daily record log from the Ames Company for $1.00, which also provides some good material for learning. (Write to Dept. JRP, Ames Division, Miles Laboratories, Inc., 1127 Myrtle St., Elkhart, Ind 46515, and ask for the Clinilog.)

Home Blood Sugar Testing

It's clear that we strongly recommend this method of testing to see if blood sugar is high, low, or normal. There can be no secrets, no relying on "hunches" as to what's going on inside your child's body. It makes sense if you have a newly diagnosed diabetic baby to start off the proper way.

What's more, many doctors predict that in a few years, urine testing will be a thing of the past.

There are four ways to test for blood sugar at home. The preferred method for insulin-dependent diabetics is to use one of the following products:

Dextrostix Reagent Strips   Choose a finger on your baby's hand—the thumb and little finger tend to bleed more freely. Hold the hand under warm water a few seconds because a warm finger bleeds more easily than a cold one. Swab the site with alcohol and blow the alcohol dry (pricking on dry alcohol hurts less than wet). Prick the finger with a lancet or an Autolet and squeeze out a large drop of blood. Touch the blood to the pad on the chemically treated plastic Dextrostix, wait sixty seconds, then wash the blood off the strip with running tap water or with a plastic squeeze bottle. Pat the strip dry with tissue or a piece of cotton.

Compare the color with the chart given on the bottle. If the child has no glucose in his blood, the color should be cream; 25 mg. of glucose should give you a moss green; 45 mg. should give you a bluish-green; 90 mg. should give you teal blue; 130 mg. is sapphire blue; 175 mg. is dark midnight blue; 250 mg. or more will show a purplish-blue. You can cut the strips in half (lengthwise) for economy purposes and they even require a smaller drop of blood, that way.

Chemstrip bg   These are also chemically treated plastic strips with a color chart printed on the container. You put a drop of your child's blood on the strip, wait sixty seconds, wipe the blood off with cotton (not rough tissues, which may strip off the chemical), wait another sixty seconds, then compare colors. (It should be stressed that this test can be easily misread by an adult patient who is having an insulin reaction and whose visual acuity and possible confusion may throw him off.)

Visidex Reagent Strips   This is the newest product, developed by Ames, which also employs a color chart for visual interpretation of blood sugar results. It takes about sixty to ninety seconds and has a single color comparison plan—there's no need to interpret two different colors simultaneously.

Electronic Meters for Reading Blood   For absolute accuracy, it's now possible to have, in your home, a blood-reading meter that gives you an exact reading of the blood sugar. This is not only wonderful for color-blind people, it's wonderful for anybody! Although they're expensive (about $340 the last time we looked), they are tax-deductible with a doctor's prescription.

The Ames Company of Elkhart, Indiana, and the Bio-Dynamics Company of Indianapolis, Indiana, put out various versions of these so-called reflectance colormeters that give regular or digital readings depending on the model.*

There is one other test that you should know about—the Glycohemoglobin Test or Hemoglobin Alc. This is the measurement of your baby's blood sugar that, by showing the amount of glucose clinging to individual cells, also shows the child's stage of general control over the last two or three months.

It should be done in a laboratory every three or four months, and has already been described more fully in the section outlining the minimal examination your child requires after diagnosis (see pp. 13–14).

What's a Good Blood Sugar Reading? It differs from person to person and you and your doctor ought to determine, together, what blood sugar readings you should be aiming for. In order to help you judge, here's a chart that was published in the magazine *Diabetes Care* which provides a *range* of blood sugars from ideal to acceptable. It's important to remember that ideal blood sugar goals are not immutable standards that everyone with diabetes ought to aim for. For some people, less perfect goals may be more appropriate to that person's particular body and psychological chemistry.

Blood Sugar Target Levels*

BLOOD SUGARS

	Ideal	Acceptable
Fasting	60-90 mg/dl	60-130 mg/dl
Before meals	60-105 mg/dl	60-130 mg/dl
After meals (1h)	140 mg/dl or less	180 mg/dl or less
After meals (2h)	120 mg/dl or less	150 mg/dl or less

* From Skyler, J., Skyler, D., Seigler, D. E. et al. Algorithms for adjustment of insulin dosage by patients who monitor blood glucose. *Diabetes Care,* 1981, 4, pp. 311-18.

BUT HOW DO YOU GET THEM TO SIT STILL?

Precious little has been written about the logistics of getting that squirming, screaming baby on your lap to sit still for his blood test or injection. There is no question that the attitudes developed by these littles closely correspond to parental attitudes. If you think your infant can't sense when

*Note that Dextrostix users must use the Dextrometer or the Glucometer put out by Ames.

you cringe before you prick his finger, you're wrong. He can. So the first thing to do is to calm yourself—and you do that by having experience. You give anyone who will sit still for them shots of sterile water, blood tests, finger jabs until you feel comfortable with the idea of (1) sharp things, and (2) blood. The faster you come to accept the things you have to do in a *casual* (not careless) manner, the faster your little diabetic will fall into that attitude also. It always helps to hear how others manage, so read on.

David G.:

The hardest thing I ever had to do in my life was to stick an insulin needle, or even a blood-letting lancet, into that tiny arm. A one-year-old doesn't have so much tissue and you feel like it's ripping when the point goes in. But, like everything else, you do get used to it. How we handle it is to simply try to distract her each time: it's hard to reason or explain to a baby with a twelve-word vocabulary. My wife gives her lipstick to hold, a pail of water to mush in, pots and pans to bang on—something fun and distracting. I think that the point is to just get the damned thing OVER with. After you've done it about twenty dozen times, the baby hardly notices. As she gets older, we'll have her take more of an active role.

Anne F.:

It gets easier, a little bit anyway, no kidding, as they get older. My son is two and a half and we make a game of the whole thing. We inject—rather, he does it—a rubber doll with "skin" that "gives" much like human skin.* Or we take "blood samples" from a Teddy, or a ball, or an orange—whatever he chooses. Sometimes he chooses me. That's all right, too. He has one job now: to put on the alcohol and blow it dry. As he gets older, he'll do more for himself.

Simon:

My four-year-old daughter gives my wife a much harder time than she gives me. That's because my wife plays a no-win game: she chases my daughter all over the house, involves herself in screaming and verbal battles, and *negotiates* each finger prick as if my daughter's doing *her* a big favor. Seems to me that she gives a shot of anxiety along with each shot of insulin. I surely don't know all the answers, but I think an attitude of "Okay, this is for *you,* I know it's not terrific but let's do it and get it over with" works

*You can use any rubber doll, or write to a company called Sugar Babe, P.O. Box 3133, Princeton, NJ 08540, for a doll especially designed for the purpose.

better. I never chase after her. The decisions about which site to use, when to do the prick, all those are the child's decisions.

Marjorie L.:

My six-year-old has to practically lie on my baby so I can give her a shot. One day, the six-year-old said to me: "Mommy, you're squeezing her arm so hard—that's why she's crying." When I looked, I saw my baby's arm was red where I was clutching her. My own hatred of that damn needle was coming through as clear as day to her. When I learned to relax and accept it, she did. She really did.

THE EMERGENCIES

Despite the best of precautions on your part, despite the most meticulous care, there may still come times when your baby needs emergency care. These are the scary times and they try men's (also women's) souls. They're no one's fault—that's the first thing to remember—it's just the nature of the illness.

The Insulin Reaction: Stage One

Insulin reactions are also known as *hypoglycemia* and they come on FAST—within minutes or a few hours. They occur when the blood sugar drops very rapidly because the balance between insulin and sugar is upset. Watch for it most frequently

- after excessive physical activity
- if the baby fails to eat the proper amount at the proper time
- if you've injected too much insulin.

Older children and adults often can sense a reaction coming on because they may feel sweaty, faint, trembly, cranky; they may have a racing pulse or cold skin. While infants and toddlers probably sense the same thing, they're not so terrific at telling you what's happening because of their thirty-seven-word or less vocabulary. Therefore, they react by acting cranky, irrational, or otherwise just *different.* One mother says her child always gets the same "crazy-looking expression on his face"; another says her child lets out an eerie, unearthly moan. Because each child reacts differently to this low blood sugar or hypoglycemic state, you will probably come to know your own little one's special signals after a while.

The thing to do is to give sugar—fast. Orange juice, Lifesavers, a non-diet soda like Coke, all are frequently used to raise the blood sugar quickly. Monogel (manufactured by Monoject) and Glutose (manufactured by Paddock Laboratories) are other special quick sugar sources that can be carried in a pocket or purse when traveling. A small amount, such as 25 grams, can abort a reaction in most cases. It takes about ten minutes for the blood sugar to read normal; *but the symptoms may last half an hour or longer,* so don't be impatient and give horrendous amounts of sugar in your anxiety to see instant improvement.

The important thing is to get that sugar food into the child as soon as possible. But suppose the crankiness is not coming from a low blood sugar condition and is instead caused by the usual cranky baby irritants—teething, tiredness, open safety pin? What do you do if you really don't know the true cause of your baby's odd behavior? You give the sugar—that's what you do. If you were wrong, and the crankiness had nothing to do with low blood sugar, you'll see a little sugar spilled in the urine; but so what? Better to err on the side of a little extra sugar than have a full-blown insulin reaction on your hands. After this "happening" your baby may be famished, so have a regular snack handy. If you're lucky, this will be the worst of the low blood sugar emergency.

The Insulin Reaction: Stage Two

However, you're probably like the rest of us and not so lucky, all the time. Your baby may have progressed into a hypoglycemic state that is quite serious, and now it's imperative that you work really quickly to avoid any lasting damage. If the baby is unable to take regular high-sugar food because she's slipping into unconsciousness, it's crucial that you get some sugar down her anyway. Try these products, all highly recommended by JDF parents:

1. *Pancake syrup* in a spouted bottle gets that sweetness into a small mouth, safely and quickly.

2. *Instant Glucose* comes in a tube. It can be ordered from the Diabetes Association of Cleveland, 2022 Lee Road, Cleveland, Ohio 44118. (Tubes are currently $1.00 each and a minimum of three tubes has to be ordered.)

3. *Cake gel* (the same stuff you use for icing decoration on your baked goods). It comes in a tube, tastes delicious, but doesn't work quite as fast as Mono-Gel (see below).

4. *Mono-Gel,* same principle as the icing gels.

5. *A fingerful of sweet.* Actually, any jam, honey, or jelly can be smeared onto your finger and inserted between the gums and the cheek—which is the best place to put all of this stuff.

TIP: Remember to keep any gels at room temperature to avoid solidifying.

When All Else Fails, Grab the Glucagon

If it is absolutely impossible to get your baby to take sugar by mouth, or if the baby is unconscious, call your doctor. Meanwhile, inject ½cc. of a protein hormone called glucagon (Lilly) into the buttocks in order to raise the blood sugar quickly so that the baby is responsive enough to take oral sugar. Wait fifteen minutes. If there's no response, inject another ½cc. Hopefully, you will have been in contact with your doctor during this time. If you have not been able to reach the doctor and your baby is unconscious—don't wait another minute and get him to a hospital.

Things You Should Know About Glucagon:

1. It's very safe—you can't give an overdose.

2. It needs a prescription, and it goes out of date, so make sure you have some up-to-date glucagon in the house *at all times.*

3. The sooner that glucagon is administered after an insulin reaction starts, the better its chance of working.

4. It takes fifteen minutes to work. (It really does, so even if you're a mental wreck, be patient.)

5. Don't prepare the glucagon for injection until you actually need it, but make sure you've read the instructions in the kit *before* an emergency arises to familiarize yourself with them.

6. Glucagon is injected in the same way insulin is injected.

7. Glucagon only acts for a limited time, so make sure you feed the baby as soon as she awakens and can safely swallow (sugarwater, Coke, orange juice, at first; and then a long-lasting carbohydrate source like a cracker, muffin, or bread).

8. If your child should vomit as she wakes up, turn her to one side and put her face down. That position is best to avoid the aspiration of stomach contents into the lungs.

9. Glucagon can be stored at room temperature.

TIP: If your child is to be left with a sitter, grandparents, or neighbor, it is a great advantage to choose someone who knows how to administer an injection of glucagon, which should always be on hand at home.

The Diabetic Coma

This is the other side of the coin from the insulin reaction, and it comes from too much sugar and not enough insulin. Unlike the insulin reaction, it comes on slowly and is really easy to miss because it progresses, over a period of hours, days, or even weeks. Watch for it when

- you've injected too little insulin
- the baby has gone off her diet
- the baby is sick with a cold, infection, virus, fever
- the baby is *very* unhappy and suffering from severe emotional stress. (We've heard stories of babies being left for long periods of time with strange or unfriendly babysitters and they have developed high blood sugar. This does *not* mean you would not leave your child with sitters; it only means that you choose your babysitters with care.)

How can you tell if a diabetic coma is looming? The signs are increased thirst and urination, large amounts of sugar in the blood or ketones in the urine, loss of appetite, nausea or vomiting, weakness, abdominal pains, and assorted aches and pains.

What to do about it? First of all, call the doctor. The child, in the meantime, would be kept warm and quiet in bed, fed fluids without sugar, and tested, as usual. Remember: it may sound strange but you do not have to be unconscious to be in a diabetic coma.

Insulin reaction and diabetic coma are the two most serious emergencies. Sometimes, an emergency room is the best place to go for a severe insulin reaction and it's the ONLY place to go for a diabetic coma. But— believe it or not—there are some emergency rooms in hospitals that have done more damage to diabetic children than good because the personnel did not know any better. Before we go on to the other emergencies that may arise in your life, let's stop a moment to tell you what should and what should not happen in an emergency room. One knowledgeable JDF father actually tore the intravenous glucose equipment out of his child's arm when placed there by a harried intern who could not tell the difference between a diabetic coma (which the child had) and an insulin reaction (which the parent definitely knew his child was *not* having).

According to Dr. Henry Dolger, Professor Emeritus of Medicine at Mt. Sinai School of Medicine and Consultant for Diabetes at the Mount Sinai Hospital in New York, the following symptoms indicate *a diabetic coma (or an advanced state of keto-acidosis—the step before coma):*

You will probably have diagnosed it yourself, and the doctor should be able instantly to do so because of any or all of these signals:

- fruity odor on the breath, which indicates the presence of acetones in the bloodstream
- the presence of ketones in the urine
- a state of dehydration (the skin appears very limp, it can almost be pulled up like wax); the tongue is dry

- the eyeballs of the patient feel soft
- the patient is sometimes semi-stuporous, vomiting, weak
- the condition came on relatively slowly.

What Should Happen: Accepted Hospital Procedure

Dr. Julio Santiago, Associate Professor of Pediatrics at the St. Louis Children's Hospital in Missouri, suggests the following emergency procedures when a child is brought to a hospital in DKA (diabetic keto-acidosis). Four possible problems must be looked for and treated. They are

- dehydration
- electrolyte abnormalities
- acidosis
- associated infections.

Dehydration The loss of body water is the first thing that must be compensated for, and the child should be placed immediately on intravenous fluid like a saline solution. The amount of fluid given over the first twenty-four hours should be about 10 to 15 percent of the patient's total weight. If the child is a teenager, for example, and weighs 50 kilograms (about 110 pounds), he should receive 5 to 7 liters of fluid during the first twenty-four hours. These fluids are started often *immediately* upon making the diagnosis and are discontinued after the child is able to eat and keep down fluids.

Electrolyte Abnormalities Electrolytes are chemical substances, like potassium, which may fall to dangerous levels in the body during the course of therapy even though they are often elevated on admission. Therefore, the blood sugar tests will have to be performed at least every two hours, at first, and less frequently after the child has improved, to watch these levels very carefully.

Acidosis This is a condition caused by too much sugar and too little insulin in the bloodstream. Various methods can be used to reduce high blood sugar. Some involve continuous doses of insulin given intravenously, while others involve one- or two-hour insulin injections given subcutaneously (under the skin). The amount of insulin given will be determined by the frequent blood sugar tests that should be performed, but generally speaking, the goal during the first twelve to twenty-four hours is to lower the sugar to a value somewhere between 100 to 250 mg. per deciliter.

One of the main risks during this recovery from diabetic keto-acidosis and hyperglycemia is the development of hypoglycemia (low blood sugar).

Therefore, when the blood glucose falls to a level of 200 to 300 mg. per deciliter, glucose is added to the intravenous fluids. When the child is able to eat normally, he's transferred to routine insulin injections. Here's something else to watch for: the presence of acidosis causes a child to breathe rapidly and so become unable to empty the stomach. For this reason, especially with unconscious children, a tube is sometimes placed into the stomach to prevent the child from aspirating the contents. To monitor the acidosis, it is also sometimes necessary to get blood samples directly from an artery because the measurements of the severity of the acidosis are best done on the artery rather than the vein. These tests are especially common during the first six to twelve hours of therapy; as the child improves, so will the breathing, the ability to keep food down, and the amount of fluid in the system.

Associated Infections Fifty or more percent of children with diabetic keto-acidosis will have an associated infection such as strep throat, flu, an ear infection, or a urinary tract infection. Tests to see if these exist are considered during the first few hours after admission if there is any suspicion that one exists. In a few cases, X-rays of the chest and even a spinal tap may be needed. If the child, for instance, has a high fever and he's rundown, the doctor can't be sure, without testing, whether it's the acidosis or meningitis that's causing the fever. Throat tests and urine cultures should be taken, because if pneumonia or meningitis is present and left untreated, the result could be lethal. And, as Dr. Santiago phrases it, "most physicians consider that a high index of suspicion is warranted to rule out a serious infection." Sometimes, for every case of infection found, says the doctor, you have to screen out four or five patients who have no associated infection. But the tests are absolutely warranted, "if you're doing things right."

If you live in an area where no doctor highly skilled in diabetes management is present when your child is brought to the hospital in or near diabetic coma, the guidelines just given should be presented to the doctor in charge of your child's case. Any physician worth his salt will not mind considering the recommendations of a specialist.

How long should it take? Improvement should be noted within a few hours, after emergency measures and diagnostic tests have been taken.

For a severe insulin reaction:
You will probably have also diagnosed this yourself because of any or all of these signals:

- the speed with which it came on
- the *lack* of a fruity acetone smell

• limpness, sweating, various states of unconsciousness, pounding of heart, trembling, irritability, irrationality.

What should happen:

NO TIME MUST BE WASTED before the child is given intravenous glucose. Improvement should be noted in a minute or so.

There are other emergencies that you should be prepared for, just in case. Some JDF parents have told us that they've managed to slip through without having to face any of these difficult situations, but they've also felt good that they were emotionally and intellectually ready should the emergencies arise.

The Throwing-Up Virus

It is essential that little ones taking insulin eat. Therefore, when any illness includes vomiting, special measures must be taken.

We offer suggestions from three diabetes specialists on what to do in this kind of emergency. Dr. Julio Santiago says that in his diabetes center, the patient gets "one free vomit." The second time the child vomits, regardless of how he feels, blood sugar must be monitored very frequently and the doctor *must* be called. A liquid diet is then prescribed (to replace the lost fluids) that includes things like jello, Seven-Up, and Gatorade.

Remember, says Dr. Santiago, that appendicitis still occurs in diabetics and is a frequent cause of abdominal pain and vomiting in the diabetic. Persistent vomiting, especially when accompanied by pain, needs immediate medical attention.

Dr. Henry Dolger suggests that all foods and liquids be withheld for at least an hour after a child first vomits. Giving food or even ginger ale immediately after such an episode is comparable to putting an ash in an eye that's already irritated—it only makes things worse. If the baby does not vomit again after waiting an hour, it's reasonably safe to start giving tiny sips of regular Coke or ginger ale, which act as antiemetics and also provide the needed carbohydrate food value. If, however, the child vomits more than once, advises Dr. Dolger, "Don't waste time playing around in an attempt to stop it." An injection of Compazine or Tigan (check the doses with your doctor—the smaller the child, the lesser the dose, is the rule) should be given immediately, and it's usually quite effective. (Note: Compazine and Tigan injections also control diarrhea.)

If nothing helps, the physician must be immediately consulted. Your child might need an intravenous feeding of glucose or a saline solution.

Dr. Alicia Schiffrin cautions that vomiting is so often associated with low blood sugar that people may forget it is also a symptom of the start of diabetic keto-acidosis, and that is why your physician should be notified immediately. Never stop giving your child his/her insulin dosage, says Dr. Schiffrin, but give *only* regular insulin now—never long-acting. And, she also reminds the reader, always check for acetones in the urine when a child is ill and vomiting.

—If the glucose is high and there are acetones in the urine, call your doctor right away.

—If the glucose is high and there are no acetones in the urine, keep testing for acetones and adjust the insulin dose to lower the glucose.

—If the glucose is low and there are acetones in the urine, it means that the glucose is too low and the patient probably needs more sugar (either sugar with fluid, or, if vomiting persists, an intravenously administered glucose in the hospital).

—If the urine is negative and there are no acetones and there is a normal blood sugar reading, you're home free.

NOTE: Always keep Compazine or Tigan suppositories in the house and check to see if your doctor wishes you to use them. They don't work as fast as the injectable version but they're effective and safe.

What if your child is having attacks of diarrhea, along with or separate from vomiting? Call the doctor, advises Dr. Schiffrin. "There may be at least a thousand reasons for diarrhea." If you choose to deal with it initially yourself, a mild anti-diarrhea substance like Kaopectate can be tried. Lomotil, which is available only upon prescription, has an opiate in it and can also cause severe constipation.

Discuss the possibilities of vomiting and diarrhea *before* they occur as well as while they are occurring. It does wonders for the peace of mind to know how to face the dilemma of giving your child something that won't upset the stomach but will still offer enough carbohydrates to ward off an insulin reaction. Be forewarned and have alternative possibilities all ready to try. Know what kinds of insulin adjustments you'll have to make during a sick day episode, also.

Convulsions

Dr. Robert M. Selig, a pediatric juvenile diabetes specialist from Philadelphia, describes a convulsion in this way: "When blood sugar gets really low and the brain has difficulty functioning, electrical impulses misfire and *voilà* —a convulsion!"

What are the signs? They vary, says Dr. Selig, from a mother saying on the phone that "my kid is acting funny" to delirious behavior, saying wild things, shaking all over, trembling, eyes rolling back in the head, and other bizarre actions. A real convulsion is actually a shaking episode, says Dr. Selig, but the child may be shaking from a bad reaction and not a convulsion at all. If it's a reaction or a hypoglycemic convulsion, the antidote is, of course, sugar in some form. If it's a true convulsion, and you either have doubts as to what kind it is or cannot get sugar into him—get him to a hospital immediately. It's quite rare and you'll know it because the child does not respond to sugar or glucagon injections. The hospital is necessary because the convulsion may cause the child to aspirate the contents of his stomach which, in turn, may obstruct the air passageways and hinder breathing.

The Somogyi Effect

It sounds like a science fiction movie but it's very real. All insulin-taking diabetics experience low blood sugar from time to time, and because we, as parents, have been trained to think of high blood sugar as the primary problem, we often accept frequent insulin reactions that are not too terrible as inevitable to proper control. A bad mistake. Not only are insulin reactions not terrific because of their immediate effects, but they're undesirable because they lead to a rebound of high blood sugar by what is known as the *Somogyi effect*, named after the man who discovered it. Low blood sugar initiates a release of counter-regulatory hormones, which shoot sugar very high. As a result, children who have frequent insulin reactions also have frequent high blood sugar incidents. It becomes a destructive pattern that can't be stopped until the control of sugar is stabilized. If you don't report the insulin reactions to your doctor and he keeps seeing high blood sugar test results, he'll naturally make the mistake of raising instead of lowering insulin doses—putting your baby into a vicious cycle pattern. So don't ignore insulin reactions, even if they're not bad ones.

Different doctors prescribe different treatments to cut the cycle of low blood sugar giving rise to high blood sugar and back again. Dr. Richard Bernstein of the New York Medical College, Westchester County Medical Center, Valhalla, New York, author of the ground-breaking *Diabetes: The Glucograf Method for Normalizing Blood Sugar*, says that the most common cause of the Somogyi effect is the administration of too much food or the wrong kind of food. He suggests a chewable hard candy or table sugar to reverse hypoglycemia in half an hour or less. Particularly effective, he says, is a product called Dextrosol, available in England, Canada, and Europe at candy and drug counters, and in this country by writing to the

Sugar-Free Center for Diabetics, 5623 Matilija Avenue, Van Nuys, California 91401. (Five packages sell for $2.50 postpaid, and discounts are available on large orders.)

Dr. Robert Kaye, Professor and chairman of the Department of Pediatrics at Hahnemann Medical College and Hospital of Pennsylvania, suggests that reduction of the insulin dosage will be effective in restoring stability. The Somogyi effect is instrumental in creating the "brittle" diabetics, says Dr. Kaye—those who alternate between acidosis and hypoglycemia all too often. The Somogyi effect can be suspected when a "brittle" diabetic apparently requires an unusually large dose of insulin (greater than 0.4 U/kg. in the young child).

To sum up, let's look at a chart of all these common emergencies and what to do about them.

Have It on Hand!

Finally, nothing's worse than running out of a crucial item in an emergency. Play it safe and always have all these things within easy access in your home. If they have expiration dates, make sure each item is current and ready for use:

- An extra supply of insulin
- Extra syringes
- Injectable glucagon
- Tubes of Instant Glucose, Mono Gel, cake gels, honey in a bottle with a spout, and other easy-to-get-down sugar products
- Bottles of non-diet Coca-Cola
- Injectable Compazine or Tigan (these are the antihistamines that work very fast during a throwing-up virus to sedate the brain's vomiting center)
- Compazine suppositories
- Emergency telephone numbers. In emergencies you must work hand in hand with your doctor to administer the proper amounts of food, liquid, and insulin—particularly if keto-acidosis is detected.

ALL ABOUT INSULIN

As the name implies, all insulin-dependent diabetics (and that includes juvenile-onset diabetics) need insulin to survive. That's not a whole lot of fun to contemplate but it's no reason to despair, either. Think of the alternative, which is what you'd be faced with had your child been born before insulin came onto the scene in 1921. Neither you nor your child will ever

Emergencies—Take Your Pick!

TYPE	CAUSES	SYMPTOMS	WHAT TO DO
INSULIN REACTION			
Stage One	Too much insulin Too little food Too much exercise Delayed meal	Sweaty, cranky, trembly, racing pulse, cold skin Irrational actions	Give sugar—candy, non-diet soda, orange juice, cake, honey, Monogel, glucose tablets. (Squeeze substances like honey between cheek and gum)
Stage Two		Close to unconsciousness or actually unconscious, irrational	Give instant glucose or glucagon injection. Call police or ambulance and take child to hospital emergency room
DIABETIC COMA (Keto-acidosis)	Not enough insulin Failure to follow diet (an overload of carbohydrates) Illness Emotional stress	Excessive thirst and urination Sugar and ketones in urine Aches, pains, weakness Vomiting Unconsciousness	Call doctor! Call police or emergency ambulance to take child to hospital emergency room. Meanwhile, keep child warm and in bed; give fluids without sugar if child is conscious and able to swallow

TYPE	CAUSES	SYMPTOMS	WHAT TO DO
THROWING-UP VIRUS	Illness Food doesn't agree	Vomiting, sometimes diarrhea or fever	If child vomits more than once, call doctor. Have child chew on ice, give small sips of Coke or Coke syrup. Give Compazine or Tigan injections or suppositories (per doctor's instructions). Consult with doctor regularly to see if injections of *regular* insulin should be adjusted. Check for ketones in urine, often. Sometimes it's necessary to admit child to hospital to re-stabilize him, if vomiting was severe
CONVULSIONS	Low blood sugar Other illnesses or trauma	Shaking Delirium Incoherent speech, eyes rolling back in head	Give sugar or glucagon injection. If child does not respond almost immediately, get him to hospital
SOMOGYI Effect	Experts differ: some say too much insulin; others say too much or wrong kind of food	Vicious cycle of low to high to low to high, etc., blood sugar	If high blood sugar *regularly* appears after low blood sugar count, discuss with doctor. Reduction of insulin dose is often prescribed. Try chewable hard candy like Dextrosol or Lifesavers to reverse hypoglycemia if cause is too much or wrong kind of food

learn to *love* the shots (and it's not the same as being dependent on food and water for life, no matter what the Pollyannas would tell you), but if your attitude is accepting and businesslike, your child's will surely be similar.

What does insulin do, anyway? The body's cells rely on a fuel known as glucose. Glucose is manufactured from the various foods in our diet and transported to the cells via the inland waterway called the bloodstream. But in order to fire that fuel into the cells, a spark is required. That spark is insulin, a hormone manufactured in the beta cells of the pancreas gland. Because your child is not manufacturing his/her own insulin sparks, the glucose cannot be fired up into the cells of the body. Therefore, you must give the spark by injection. In the United States, insulin today is available and prescribed in U-100 strength. Something to remember is this: a unit of insulin is always the same, no matter what strength you use (in other countries, insulin is still prescribed in different strengths).

Kinds of Insulin

For the first time, diabetics really have alternative choices in the variety and strength of the insulin they will use. Until recently, there was only one kind of insulin, the regular or fast-acting, and it required multiple injections to carry one through the day. Now, there are longer-acting insulins which, when injected just once or twice, are able to shoot off at various times during the day, eliminating the need for many shots.

Naturally, as with everything else, there is controversy on this kind of insulin. The positive argument is that the longer-acting insulin keeps your child covered throughout the day and even the night. The negative side is that some laypeople and physicians are very wary of the longer-acting insulins because they feel it's unnatural for the body to have to sustain large amounts of insulin for long periods of time. When a non-diabetic person eats a piece of candy, his pancreas gives off just a few units of insulin to help the cells metabolize the sugar. There is never a huge amount of insulin circulating throughout the body. When a diabetic person takes a long-acting insulin, if there are not enough carbohydrates in the body for the injected amount to work on, the extra insulin keeps circulating in the body, nevertheless. Small children and adults are equally tied into a certain amount of food and exercise once they've taken that shot.

Dr. Julio Santiago says: "The primary goal of giving insulin is to replace it in a natural or a physiologic pattern. Originally when insulin was discovered in 1921, and the first patients were started in 1922, the only insulin available was short-acting insulin. Therefore, all patients were on short-acting insulin and, usually, three to four injections a day. With the development of the longer-acting insulin, it now became possible to treat diabetes not with three or four but with one injection of insulin a day.

"However, it's been clear for the last ten to fifteen years that in some ways, in some aspects, the longer-acting insulins are a mixed blessing because they do not permit the diabetic to have the normal fluctuations in the levels of insulin that they would have if they were not diabetic. And all you get is a big tide of insulin, rather than the increases at suppertime and the low level between meals. So multiple insulin injections were rediscovered in the seventies, when it became possible to let the patient monitor his own blood sugar and to train him to interpret the findings on a daily basis so he could adjust his own insulin. The new regimens involve multiple shots, mostly of short-acting insulin before meals, and minimizing the use of long-acting insulin. This trend is continuing into the eighties and, I think, can be expected to continue until we find a workable transplant or cure for diabetes."

To be very fair, there are surely many doctors who don't buy this theory at all, and who feel that long-acting insulin is the greatest boon in modern diabetes research. Most doctors today prescribe a combination of the types of insulin. Again, you *do* have a choice, and that's why it's better to be a diabetic today than at any other time in history. Discuss the alternatives with your physician, then decide together on the best approach for your child. To help you make an informed choice, a breakdown of what's available follows.

Insulin Rates

1. *Rapid-acting* is also known as *regular (R)*. The insulin takes about thirty minutes to go into effect and it's this insulin you use in an emergency. It can be given intravenously for faster action.

2. *Intermediate action* insulin begins to work about two to four hours after the injection and lasts from fourteen to twenty-four hours.

3. *Prolonged action or Long-acting insulin* takes from four to eight hours to begin action and can last from twelve hours to two days.

Key Words to Understanding the Following Insulin Chart

Onset—how long the insulin takes to start working

Peak—when the insulin reaches its top effect

Duration—the amount of hours the insulin works to lower your blood sugar

Appearance—what the insulin looks like—is it cloudy or clear?

Insulins Currently Available in the United States and Canada

TYPE OF INSULIN	ONSET OF ACTIVITY (HOURS)	PEAK OF ACTIVITY (HOURS)	DURATION OF ACTIVITY (HOURS)	MANUFACTURER & BRAND NAME	ANIMAL SOURCE	PURITY (ppm) < = less than > = greater than	APPEARANCE
RAPID-ACTING							
Regular (R)	½	2½-5	6-8	Lilly: Iletin I†	Beef/Pork	< 50ppm	clear
				Iletin II	Beef	< 10	
				Iletin II†	Pork	< 10	
				Squibb-Novo: Improved Insulin*	Pork	< 25	
				Purified Insulin*	Pork	< 10	
	½-1	2-3	5-7	Squibb-Novo: Actrapid	Pork	< 1	
				Nordisk: Velosulin	Pork	< 10	
				Connaught: Insulin Toronto†	Beef/Pork	> 50	
					Pork	> 50	
					Beef	> 50	
Semilente (S)	1-2	5-10	16	Lilly: Iletin I†	Beef/Pork	< 50	cloudy
				Squibb-Novo: Improved Insulin*	Beef	< 25	
				Squibb-Novo: Semitard	Pork	< 1	
	½-1	5-8	12-16	Connaught: Semilente†	Beef/Pork	> 50	
Sulphated Insulin	½-1	2-3	5-7	Connaught: Sulphated Insulin†	Beef	> 50	
INTERMEDIATE-ACTING							
NPH (N)	1½	8	24	Lilly: Iletin I†	Beef/Pork	< 50	cloudy
				Iletin II	Beef	< 10	
				Iletin II†	Pork	< 10	
				Squibb-Novo: Improved Insulin*	Beef	< 25	
				Purified Insulin*	Beef	< 10	
				Squibb-Novo: Protaphane NPH	Pork	< 1	
				Nordisk: Insulatard	Pork	< 10	
	1-3	6-12	18-28	Connaught: NPH Insulin†	Beef/Pork	> 50	
					Pork	> 50	
					Beef	> 50	

Type	Onset	Peak	Duration	Brand	Source	Purity (ppm)	Appearance
70% NPH/ 30% Regular	½	2&8	24	Nordisk: Mixtard	Pork	< 10	cloudy
Lente (L)	2-4	8	24	Lilly: Iletin I†	Beef/Pork	< 50	
				Iletin II	Beef	< 10	
				Iletin II†	Pork	< 10	
				Squibb-Novo: Improved Insulin*	Beef	< 25	
				Purified Insulin*	Beef	< 10	
				Squibb-Novo: Monotard	Pork	< 1	
				Lentard	Beef/Pork	< 1	
	1-3	6-12	18-28	Connaught: Lente†	Beef/Pork	> 50	
					Pork	< 50	
LONG-ACTING							
Protamine Zinc (P) (PZI)	4-8	12-24	36	Lilly: Iletin I†	Beef/Pork	< 50	cloudy
				Iletin II	Beef	< 10	
				Iletin II	Pork	< 10	
	3-7	15-22	24-36	Connaught: PZI Insulin†	Beef/Pork	> 50	
Ultralente (U)	4-8	16	36	Lilly: Iletin I†	Beef/Pork	< 50	cloudy
				Squibb-Novo: Improved Insulin*	Beef	< 25	
				Squibb-Novo: Ultratard	Beef	< 1	
	5-8	16-24	28-36	Connaught: Ultralente†	Beef/Pork	> 50	

† Available in Canada

* Prior to January 1982, all Squibb insulin contained both beef and pork insulin and had a purity of approximately 10,000 ppm. Their newer, purer products include the words "Improved" or "Purified" on the label.

Reproduced with the permission of the Juvenile Diabetes Foundation. We have added a seventh category, Appearance.

Remember that the numbers you see under the headings on this and other charts in other books are only *average* numbers. Insulin works differently on different people; indeed, its activity varies from person to person in every aspect and even from day to day in the same person. It's maddening, sure, but eventually your child's individual experiences will help you and your doctor to make adjustments in your own personal dosage.

A Few Notes About Insulin

—Insulin is collected from the pancreases of cows and pigs; today, usually most forms are a combination of both. An exciting development is the biosynthetically produced *human insulin,* discussed more fully in Chapter 5.

—Wouldn't it be easier to take it by mouth? Sure, but you can't. Digestive juices from the body soon destroy insulin when administered by mouth, so it must be injected directly into the bloodstream via the skin (subcutaneously).

—Can you have an insulin allergy? Yes. Sometimes it goes away. Sometimes a *pure* beef or pork insulin can be used with greater success. Sometimes a person with diabetes has to undergo desensitization by taking progressively greater amounts of the insulin concentration, as hay fever patients desensitize themselves against pollen. Luckily, the newer, highly purified insulins that are available today have reduced the incidence of these allergic reactions.

—What are those funny depressions I sometimes see in the skin of insulin users? Some people do develop a wasting of the fat tissue just below the surface of the skin, called *atrophy.* Alternating injection sites seem to help this problem, which is luckily less frequent with the advent of the newer, purer insulin. Injecting insulin at room temperature often helps the atrophy problem. Try, also, injecting the pure pork insulin directly into the atrophied site.

Hypertrophy, the buildup of fat tissue at the injection site, is also not seen as readily with the newer insulins.

Prepare for—Injection

(Instructions for use of disposable syringes; why would anybody use the other?)

1. Wash your hands (a nice touch), roll the insulin bottle between your palms to warm and mix it. (Check the bottle to make sure the expiration date has not come and that the top of the bottle is in perfect condition.

Damaged bottles and expired insulin can always and should always be returned for proper credit.) Never use insulin that has been frozen or heated.

2. Remove the cap from the insulin bottle and clean rubber stopper with an alcohol swab: do NOT remove the stopper.

3. Select a site and swab it with alcohol.

4. Draw the plunger back to the mark on the syringe that tells you your appropriate dose of insulin. This fills the space with air. Why do you need air? It's the same principle as when you punch two holes in a juice can: air must go in one hole for the juice to pour easily out the other.

5. Next, insert the needle through the rubber stopper and inject the air into the insulin bottle.

6. Turn the bottle upside down without removing the needle. Pull the plunger back *just beyond* the mark showing your correct dose.

7. Now, push the plunger *slowly* back to the exact mark of your dose. This should get rid of any air bubbles. (If bubbles persist, gently tap syringe barrel.)

8. Remove the needle from the bottle stopper. Be careful you don't change the plunger position.

Prepare for—Injection of Two Mixed Insulins

Your doctor will give you exact instructions as to the amounts of insulin needed. A general rule of thumb for infants is to use a small amount of NPH to tide them over the night along with small amounts of regular insulin. Toddlers often have a ratio of almost equal parts of NPH and regular insulin prescribed for them. This is how to prepare the mixed insulin:

1. Draw air into the syringe equal to the dosage prescribed for the intermediate-acting insulin (Lente or NPH).

2. Put the needle through the center of the Lente or NPH bottle and inject the air into it.

3. Withdraw the needle—empty.

4. Draw air into the syringe equal to the dosage prescribed for the regular insulin.

5. Push the needle through the *regular* bottle and inject the air.

6. Withdraw the needle with the proper dosage of *regular* insulin.

7. Turn the intermediate insulin bottle upside down and insert the same needle into the stopper.

8. Pull the plunger back to total the combined amount of units. You've got it!

Now—Inject!

1. Pinch a fold of flesh between two fingers on the site you've selected. Wipe the site with alcohol. Blow it dry—it will hurt less.

2. Insert the needle quickly straight in, *not at a slant,* all the way.

3. Push the plunger that injects the insulin. Some people check to see if they've hit a small blood vessel with every injection. This is *not* necessary. Do not withdraw the syringe to look for blood because this increases the trauma at the site of the injection by making the needle wobble; it just isn't important to see whether there's a drop of blood or not.

4. Release the fold of flesh, press an alcohol pad near the needle, and withdraw it. You're done!

The Automatic Injector

The Most Wonderful Invention Known to Nervous Injectees, Nervous Injectors, and Learners.

The automatic injector is wonderful for people who hate needles or blood; for children who have trouble reaching certain injection sites; for injecting with only one hand; for teaching a child to inject. It's almost painless and gives a perfect shot each time. If you decide to try one and anyone tells you you're getting your baby to rely on a "crutch" instead of facing up to the realities of his/her illness, say something nasty—even obscene—to that person and ask if ordering a pushbutton phone instead of a dialer or buying a car with an automatic drive instead of a stick shift is using a "crutch." Anything that makes a difficult business easier is a gift.

There are many models available. They range from about $60 to $100 in cost, unless you opt for the prime rib special (selling for about $800), which is an injector without needles that uses jet pressure to spray in the insulin. One of the best automatic injectors, many parents say, is the *Inject-o-matic,* just recently available from the American Medical Company (441 Flagstaff Drive, Greensbury, PA 15601). It sells for about $60, can be used with all disposable syringes, both the B-D (Becton-Dickinson) and Monoject, both 1cc. and lo-dose, which is appropriate for your baby. It doesn't hurt, there's no blood at all, and when your child is older, he/she can reach new injection sites and inject with either hand. It's small and handy to carry around. You can't even see the needle, which is a nice bonus for young children. It's both speed- and depth-controlled. Magic? No, just a big help.

There's only one negative about any automatic device: they are, in a sense, gadgets, and they do break. You really should make sure your child eventually learns to inject him/herself with a regular needle and syringe by the age of nine, even if you opt for the automatic injector most of the time. You never know when the automatic will spring a spring...

Tips and Touts About Injections

—The low dose, disposable syringes are the easiest. Get one that measures up to only 50 units (each line is 1 unit).

—The thinnest needles hurt the least: 28 gauge put out by B-D are the thinnest. These are Lo Dose needles, *created* for babies.

—The buttocks are less sensitive to pain than most other spots, and in a very young child, you'll find the most flesh there.

—Some new information on rotating sites: although we've been told for years that it's important to rotate the injection sites all over the body, Dr. Alan Rubin, Assistant Clinical Professor of Medicine at the University of San Francisco Medical College and head of the San Francisco Diabetes Medical Group, says that's now *passé*: "Contrary to decades of diabetic teaching, rotation of sites makes, we now feel, control more difficult. The uptake of insulin from varying sites is different and will change depending on the amount of exercise the diabetic opts for. Therefore, we advise patients to use only the abdomen, which provides enough sites for rotation to avoid insulin atrophy."

Again, discuss this with your doctor and use your own best judgment about rotation—after hearing all the facts. Here's some more information to help you decide. Insulin injected into the abdomen is absorbed faster than insulin injected anywhere else. Arms come next. Thin parts of the body for sites cause faster absorption than fat parts. Areas that will be well exercised cause the insulin injected there to speed up its action: a toddler who is throwing a ball with his right arm should have his injections elsewhere.

—Angle of the needle at injection? Here's some more brand-new information: despite decades of putting the needle in at an angle, diabetes authority Dr. Henry Dolger says that inserting the needle straight into the site in a perpendicular-to-the-skin position is much less painful and generally easier. Going in on an angle leaves a bump, explains Dr. Dolger. "Furthermore, if you traverse a layer of skin at a slant, you cut more nerves (making the shot more painful) than if you go straight in."

—Worried about a few bubbles in the syringe like an adolescent we know who accidentally injected himself with a whole syringe full of air? He realized with horror what he'd done, called an ambulance, and then lay down to die. Naturally, he didn't. Dr. Dolger says that injecting air bubbles under the skin is not the same as injecting air into a vein, which can be lethal. The only problem with bubbles in the syringe is that a copious amount takes up space that should be filled with insulin. Instead of 2 units of insulin, you may be getting 1 of insulin and 1 of bubbles. So be careful. But don't be terrified that you'll inject a fatal air bubble into your baby—it won't happen!

To get rid of air bubbles, hold the syringe and the bottle upside down so that the air bubbles in the syringe rise to the top of the barrel. You can tap the syringe barrel lightly to coax bubbles into the needle. Push in the plunger enough to expel the air back into the bottle. If your insulin dosage is now reading less than you need, take in some more from the bottle.

—Needle clogs? It happens. The best preventive is to complete the injection within five seconds after you've penetrated the skin. If it does clog, withdraw it, and note on a piece of paper the number of units you administered before the clogging took place. You can do this by writing down the original dose and subtracting the units remaining in the clogged syringe. Take a whole new syringe and inject only what was lost in the old one.

—Needle squirts? If you think you've lost some insulin because a bit spurted out during the injection or perhaps a bit was washed away in the blood flow, don't give your child another injection. You'd probably be arranging for an insulin reaction by doing that. Just feed him a bit less and check his blood for sugar a little sooner than you'd normally do so. If it's high, you may have to give him a small extra dose.

—Insulin should be kept in a cool place but never frozen, which ruins it. Although you might keep unopened bottles in the fridge, you don't have to refrigerate your open insulin. Room-temperature insulin is far more comfortable to receive in a shot than cold insulin and it might prevent atrophy. And never stash insulin bottles in warm places like glove compartments or on radiators. Insulin can be kept, says diabetologist Dr. Fredda Ginsburg-Fellner, for one and one half years at 80 degrees without losing its potency.

—Don't accept anything but perfect products. If the vials are broken or the NPH is flaky or the expiration date on the insulin you've just purchased is past, return it. (In a pinch, experienced doctors and parents have told us that they've safely used expired insulin. If none other is available, it can't hurt and its effectiveness will probably not be significantly diminished, although we don't advise using it if you don't have to.)

—Filling the needle. You already know how difficult it is to draw up and inject the tiny amounts necessary for infants; sometimes half units and even quarter units have to be administered. Several JDF parents find that if they put a bit of air behind the liquid, there's more to push, and it goes in much easier.

—NEVER put a needle in the inside of an arm or leg; always use the fleshy, upper, outer quadrant. Since veins and arteries are no-trespassing land, you have no worry about hitting them in these fleshy areas because the needle's too short to reach them. The idea is to get that needle just under the skin. Don't panic if you see a drop of blood on the cotton after you withdraw the needle, because tiny capillaries abound everywhere.

—You *can* reuse disposable syringes, say many parents, and at least two independent studies back them up. One study of eighteen diabetics reported in *Diabetes Care* (September/October 1979) showed that syringes can be safely reused (which saves a healthy amount of money), and another study involving thirty diabetics, reported in the *British Medical Journal* (June 2, 1979), produced similar findings. It must be said that a B-D spokesman warned of possible needle dullness, needle breakage, and blurred, worn-off measurement graduations with reuse of disposable syringes.

THE SPECIAL SITUATIONS

Having a very young child with diabetes brings out the saintly qualities—not to mention the murderous instincts—in parents. It's a challenge, no question, and once you get through these earliest years you will deserve a medal in creativity, a trip to Europe, a VERY big boat. You'll probably get none of them. What you will get is the most splendid sense of satisfaction that you've handled some times that would flatten most other people, and that you've given a head start to a kid who has a special problem for all of life, sure, but who will probably come out of it a smashing winner. Diabetics are often wonderfully competent, self-assured, independent people. Their illness has forced them to take charge and be creative, and that makes for terrific individuals.

With most learning experiences, you usually have time to get through the various stages. But in learning to be the family of a diabetic, you learn fast. You have to. While you're sitting around assimilating new information, your toddler could be glomping down the six Mounds bars you bought for yourself. And so, it's a quick jump from the shock of the diagnosis

- to the almost mourning period where you do some heavy grief work
- to the anger period when you find out your toddler is not invited next door any more because they think diabetes is catching
- to the pity period because the cutest and most lovable person in your life has a chronic disease
- to the self-pity period because the treatment of that disease is a pain in the neck

• to—hooray—normalcy, again, and everyday fun and joy and life (it comes back, we swear it!).

Yes, it comes back. But with a difference. Diabetes is now an integral part of your life and it will change things in your home. Everyone in the family will learn to make subtle shifts in priorities, diets, concerns. No longer does there have to be the strict, unyielding bans on play, diet, and sports. And the littlest diabetic can soon learn that his disease is manageable, livable with, if not lovable.

This section will answer some questions on how to make it livable with in a variety of situations.

Before I get specific, let me tell you that the general rule of thumb at this age is to try to avoid confrontations.

If you attempt some heavy discipline around mealtime, a resulting temper tantrum can really bring on an attack of hypoglycemia—and it's important, if you're looking to the long run, to avoid these complication-producing situations. So, you try to cool it with your sugar baby, and, as the teenage vernacular would have it, you try to mellow out. It's not desperately important that Alexander learns not to empty out the pots and pans closet, especially if he's doing it at lunchtime. This is *not* to say that all discipline should be postponed until the kid's thirty-two. On the contrary, if your toddler senses you're terrified of his disease and of him, it could have some pretty serious implications for your future relationships. Young children need a firm hand in there, teaching, structuring, directing. The point is to try to be creative in that structuring, rather than authoritarian, because you really don't want to get involved in the emotional face-downs which can have direct consequences for the child's diabetes.

Actually, this is a lovely stage to watch. Your child is testing the water, learning to walk, talk, acquire new skills. You're trying to figure out how to give him enough space to do this and still define the limits. It's one thing to learn how to be assertive; it's another thing to assert yourself out of a meal when your insulin demands food. Compromise is the magic word, even at this very young stage. A snack instead of the whole meal, say, and perhaps a snack of something that isn't exactly your choice. The goal—and a limited goal it is at this very young age—is to try to avoid the physical and emotional stress that contribute to hypoglycemia or hyperglycemia. And you do this by quiet reason, even if quiet reason is not exactly the script you feel like writing. Some of the special situations you will have to be aware of in these earliest years fall into the following categories:

• Eating
• Exercise

- Naps and nighttime
- Babysitters
- Sick days

Eating: It Can Eat Your Heart Out

He's got to eat. But he's not hungry, or he's cranky and he dumps his farina
on the floor. He sits at that table and he does everything but eat: he arranges his peas in a neat circle, tears up his napkin, pokes holes into the
mashed potatoes. You could die. It's one thing when a child without diabetes does that; you either make him wear his meal or wait till the next meal
when he *is* hungry. That's simply not an alternative choice with a very
young child who's had an insulin shot. And even if you haven't yet given
the shot, you *hate* to fool around with changing the dosage to fit each meal.
So you find your own tricks and routines to handle eating.

Our First Suggestion for You: Try the Reward Theory   This does not
necessarily (although it can) mean bribes, horrible as the word sounds. A
reward can be anything from a hug to a smile of approval to a present.
Actually, it's the basis of all positive behavior—you do something because
when you do it right, it feels good and you get good vibes back from the
people around you.

A kid who finishes his dinner wonderfully can get a gold star (add
enough of these up and a gift from the dime store can be a prize), a trip to a
fun place, or a half hour extra of storytime before bed . . . whatever, as long
as it's nice. Pretty soon, the recalcitrant child begins to identify eating one's
food with a nice result. Important to note that criticism or punishment is
not part of the reward game; that's a negative reinforcement and too often,
kids end up acting negatively, acting out anger as "I'll fix you" kind of
behavior.

You reward good behavior and absolutely ignore or do not reward
poor behavior. And you'd be surprised—sometimes effusive, even over-
praise sets a tone: "Oh, wonderful, fabulous you, you actually ate sixteen
stringbeans!" After a while, again, eating well becomes a habit, and the
occasional refusal of food becomes a rarity, not the norm. It won't be long
before your toddler makes a strong connection between finishing lunch and
feeling well. He will, little as he is, gradually become self-enforcing of good
eating behavior. Much praise, rewards, and reinforcement of acceptable
eating are techniques that really do work.

And Another Suggestion   Nowhere is it permanently inscribed, is it
written in stone, for instance, that there has to be a Breakfast Time, Lunchtime, Dinnertime. Some babies and small toddlers do much better with

many smallish snacks than separate sit-down meals. Finger foods are particularly attractive to the picky eater. Close your eyes to the resulting mess, if
there is one. A chunk of hamburger in the hand is more fun than one on a
fork. Wrapping finger foods creatively also makes them appealing. Hard-
boiled egg or slices of fruit hidden in shiny silver foil or plastic bags makes
them treasures because every kid loves unwrapping and discovery. Mashed
potatoes molded into a clown face with bits of vegetables for features make
mashed potatoes an *experience.* I hear what you're saying: "Lee Ducat is
trying to get me to make mealtime into an entertainment." Well, so what if
I am? Even if it goes against your moralistic grain, you really ought to try to
relax your standards a bit in the interests of making peace and nourishment
available to your child with diabetes—in these very early years. Providing
playthings and distraction during meals doesn't really set dangerous prece-
dents. When your child is nineteen, he won't need the clown face mashed
potatoes, honest. By all means, involve your toddler in the preparation of
his food and of healthy, innovative snacks. Some pointers follow:

—Try baking, stirring, decorating together—all that makes eating the product attractive.

—Frozen fruit juices shaped in the ice-cube tray with ice-cream wooden
sticks inserted are an appealing and nourishing snack.

—The same fruit juices frozen until just before solid, then scooped up into
an ice-cream cone or a pretty bowl gives juice a new look.

—Unsweetened fruit juices (apple, orange, grapefruit, grape, etc.) laced
with seltzer give just the right kick to make an alternative to the diet soda
you hate to give so much of.

—While some kids may not like cooked vegetables, *raw* carrot sticks,
cherry tomatoes, or lightly steamed vegetables (kept as a handy snack in
fridge containers) are "grown-up" hors d'oeuvres, especially when served
with a tasty yogurt or cheese dip.

—Cut-up raw fruit, chunks of natural cheese, sesame seed breadsticks are
all fine food possibilities when figured into caloric allowances.

—A word on pizza: even the youngest kid loves it. If you make your own
toasted whole-wheat pita bread or English muffin, you do away with a lot of
the empty starch and thick bread "filler" that ordinary pizza contains.

—Build tastes now. Just as candy and other pure sugar products should be
relatively taboo in your home, high salt foods are not terrific either. If you
keep salted crackers around, and heavily salted processed foods like canned

soups (which often have sugars added), your child will come to crave salt. Kids reared on low salt and *very* low sugar diets will come to reject, by taste, sweet and salty stuff.

A Serious Word About Breakfast It doesn't have to be traditional breakfast food. If breakfast is a meal your child likes, nowhere is it written that cereal, eggs, and pancakes are the order of the day, necessarily. Nutritious homemade pizzas, toasted cheese sandwiches, natural peanut butter sandwiches are just as good as a traditional breakfast. Don't be rigid; rigid rules invite defiance and cheating, and can make undesirable foods more attractive than they would be. Also about breakfasts: the best way to get your kid to eat breakfast is to sit down and eat it with her. Encourage everyone to rise and shine fifteen minutes to a half hour earlier so as to prepare and share this meal in a family way. This is a wonderful habit to develop for nutritional and for emotional reasons.

A Really Serious Word About Advertising Nothing makes a small child feel better than when he can outsmart grown-ups—and this definitely extends to the teen years and beyond. Exposing hidden, seductive, and faulty advertisement from television, fast food vendors, and street hawkers works to make the kid feel smarter than the opposition for seeing through the hype. Jane Brody of the *New York Times* recently wrote:

> When visions of sugar plums are dancing in young heads, apples and carrot sticks are less likely to start mouths watering ... when my children first started watching commercial television, we played an advertising game: Who can tell what the company is trying to get you to believe? The other day, one of my sons told me about "the Golden Griddle Breakfast," which, the ad for a brand of syrups claims, has more protein than a cereal breakfast. "They want you to think the Golden Griddle is nutritious but it's really the pancakes that have all the protein," he correctly observed.

Making the advertisers look like charlatans, exposing them for business people and not friends, is a wonderful game/lesson/life's delight that can be started very young.

It's a good idea to stay away from many of the prepared baby foods when your child is still very small because they're loaded with sugar (Tes-Tapes or Diastix can be dipped into the baby food to test the sugar content when in doubt). Home blenders can quickly prepare baby foods from the real thing, minus the chemicals and sugar, and that's much better for any baby, of course. Now there's a relatively inexpensive food mill on the market that is portable so you can take it with you when you're visiting or at a restaurant to grind up some of your own food for your baby—on the spot.

It's a small, plastic number, and the manufacturer is Bowland-Jacobs Manu-facturing Co., Spring Valley, Illinois 61362.

Often babies and children refuse to eat because their diet is so *boring.* Educate yourself and provide variety. There's a fine exchange list* for baby foods that was published in the July/August 1980 issue of *Diabetes Care* by Marian M. Benz and Elaine Kohler (back issues are available on request). They explain, for instance, that five tablespoons of dry baby rice cereal equals one bread exchange and can be substituted for a half jar of junior rice mixed with fruit—or three pretzels. And in the fruit category, ¾ cup of a can of baby apple juice can be substituted for half a jar of strained apple-sauce.

So, the eating situation *can* be handled. Even though you think it's impossible, sometimes, you must find ways to make food attractive to any child whom you've faithfully injected with insulin. And you must find ways to make him drink, like the proverbial horse at the trough, even though he's not thirsty (ice cubes on a stick are fun to suck on). And you must find ways to make the heavily sugared foods that are advertised everywhere he looks *un*attractive. It can be done.

Exercise: The Invisible Insulin

Use it or lose it. There's no question that if you don't use your body, it works far less well—and this is true for everyone. Exercise has been called the invisible insulin because it actually lowers blood sugar and reduces a need for insulin.

It also tends to keep down your cholesterol level by encouraging a substance known as your HDLs. What are HDLs?

Dr. Charles Peterson of Rockefeller University in New York explains it this way: "There are certain proteins in the blood that carry fat proteins and they're called lipoproteins. Some appear to carry the lipids *into* the cells and they're known as LDLs, VLDLs, and the intermediate density lipoprotein, IDL. Those are the bad guys. The good guys are the ones that appear to carry fat lipids out of the cells and those are HDLs (high density lipoprotein). Exercise tends to raise the HDLs—the good guys."

Regular exercise also heads off or ameliorates the blood vessel damage and other complications often seen in older diabetics. It may seem redun-dant to think about exercise for a very young child who always appears to be moving anyway. But some move more than others. In recent studies of obese children it was discovered that a lack of exercise, not an over-eating

---

*Exchange lists are foods of equivalent value, a way to substitute one food for another to add variety but still retain the same approximate calorie, carbohydrate and fat value.

problem, made them fat. Thus, it's never too young to start implanting a *habit* of regular exercise patterns. Can a one-year-old be involved in conscious exercise apart from his regular one-year-old movements? Absolutely! Have you ever seen the swimming six-month-old babies? They'll grow up to be the healthiest kids in town. Exercise is essential for the cardiovascular system, for muscle tone, and for weight control. It has a stabilizing effect on many insulin-taking diabetics, who tend to have fewer shocky experiences than non-exercisers. What's more, researchers at the Yale University School of Medicine have found that insulin sticks better to tissues in persons who exercise than in those who don't. In addition, exercisers seem to metabolize glucose better.

Here are the important things to remember about exercise and young children:

1. Only well-controlled diabetic toddlers (as well as older children and adults) should exercise. A team of researchers from the University of Düsseldorf, in Germany, found that a further rise in blood glucose and ketones occurs when poorly controlled diabetics exercise.

2. What kind of exercise? Games involving jumping, bending, stretching, and running can be devised for toddlers. Infants can be coaxed to "walk," to sit up, to stretch, by letting them grasp your fingers and giving firm, steady pulls. Being pushed in a swing is *not* exercise. Pushing a Teddy in a swing is.

3. Youngsters should get about the same exercise every day. If you're in the habit of playing in the park with your baby during the week, and the whole family just hangs out in a more sedentary fashion on weekends, the sudden lack of activity may cause unused sugar to build up.

4. Extremes of weather cause problems for babies who should exercise every day. If you're used to sunny exercise, what do you do when it rains and you're stuck inside? You compensate with indoor activity, that's what you do. The point is to develop a regular balance of diet, insulin, and activity, and to try not to have *anything* throw that balance off.

5. You know that there's a period of strenuous activity coming up? The rule of thumb is either to increase your baby's calories a lot or to decrease his/her insulin. Some doctors say the best way is to increase the food just a little and decrease the insulin just a little. Others say the best way is to leave the insulin constant and to increase calories. You can experiment, with the guidance of your physician, to see which works best for your little one.

6. When planning for strenuous activity—a day at the zoo, say, which requires a large amount of walking for your child—always plan on having a

supply of food and/or sugar with you. Extra activity without extra food can bring on an insulin reaction.

7. When is the best time for exercise with your toddler or infant? After a meal when the blood sugar is rising, rather than before a meal when the blood sugar is low.

8. Give some thought to the kind of exercise he'll be doing before you give a shot. Unless you give shots exclusively in the toddler's abdomen areas, make sure you give the injection in a part of his body that won't be heavily involved in the type of exercise you have planned. If you're doing some running exercise, the leg should not be used for an injection site. If your toddler is playing ball, stay away from his throwing arm. Increased activity causes insulin to be used up more quickly—something you'd like to avoid.

9. Keep this thought in mind: although you can't force your baby to crawl, you can make it worth his while to do so. "The more you move babies," says Dr. Peterson, "and pay attention to them, the better they grow and develop."

To sum up: Dr. Anthony Cerami, Professor of Medicine and Biochemistry at Rockefeller University in New York, says, "From a scientific point of view, the evidence that exercise is useful in diabetes control is really overwhelming!"

Naps and Nighttime

The greatest fear of many parents is that their young child will suffer an insulin reaction (hypoglycemia) during sleep and they'll have no way of knowing about it. Older children can often feel such episodes coming on and they can do something to ward it off. But even if a baby or a toddler also senses trouble, he can't communicate his discomfort. In the past, when confronted with unexplainable crankiness, sweatiness, or cold skin, parents were told to feed some sugar to the child, even if they had doubt as to the presence of low blood sugar; better to have a little spilled sugar, if wrong, than an insulin reaction. Now, with the advent of the home blood sugar monitoring, you can check out your suspicions in a moment.

Complications *can* set in during sleep time and that's why parents of children with diabetes check their sleeping kids more frequently than the parent who kisses his kid goodnight and doesn't see him till morning. Dr. Henry Dolger suggests that you pass a hand over a sleeping child's forehead for "any signs of perspiration that cannot be attributed to humidity or temperature." A clammy forehead or underarm perspiration could mean an insulin reaction; if in doubt, the child should be awakened and given fruit juice or candy. Remember that it takes ten to fifteen minutes for the blood-stream to absorb the sugar, so wait for it to take effect and don't overdose your kid with sugar in your anxiety.

On the other hand, if your toilet-trained child has wet his bed or is making too many nocturnal trips to the bathroom, or if your diaper-clad baby seems just inordinately soaked with urine, has a hot, dry forehead, and is crying for water, it may be the sign of hyperglycemia and impending ketosis. In this case, your child needs some extra regular insulin.

If your baby is in the habit of "shocking out" during sleep time, be sure to give him a snack—and that snack should be something more than milk—before sleep. This is a good routine for all diabetics to adopt.

What if you're still seeing insulin reactions during sleep at night and your baby has not had more exercise or less food than usual? If all seems status quo, you're probably giving too much intermediate-acting insulin in the morning shot. Check with your physician, who will probably advise cutting out a tiny amount of the longer-acting insulin; and then, if you see a surge of blood sugar during the day, compensate with a small extra amount of regular insulin in that morning shot.

Dr. Fredda Ginsberg-Fellner, diabetologist of the Mount Sinai Hospital in New York, agrees that the thought of a baby having a reaction in the middle of the night can be frightening. "They're prone to reactions, their brains are still growing, and it's a good idea to cut out the evening shot of insulin if your baby has frequent insulin reactions," she says. "Waking the child up for a snack before you go to bed is an absolute must, also. But don't worry," she adds. "It's been my experience that almost all babies wake up and cry out—loud enough to wake their parents—if a reaction's coming on."

Okay, the worst fear, let's get it out: Can your baby die during the night if he/she's had an insulin reaction and nobody is aware of it? In *The Diabetic's Book,* June Biermann and Barbara Toohey answer that question this way: "No doctor we've talked to has ever had a diabetic die from an insulin reaction in his or her sleep, except in one instance. The diabetic went to bed drunk and wound up literally dead drunk. What happened was that the alcohol suppressed the body's method of spontaneous recovery." Since very few toddlers have a drinking problem (alcohol, not milk), you needn't worry. Ordinarily, when the control of your child's diabetes is good, he/she will store sugar as glycogen* and that sugar will be there if your child has problems during sleep.

---

*Glucose, the end product of the body's carbohydrate metabolism, is what fuels the body, primarily. It's used immediately for energy or it's stored in the liver and muscle in the form of glycogen to be called on for energy at another time, when it's needed.

Whatever you do, do NOT get into the habit of waking yourself up several times a night to check a baby who's been tested as normal and who is having no trouble. If you think a baby can't sense the fear of parent specters hovering over him at many odd hours in the night, you're wrong. You'll make yourselves and the baby absolutely bananas if you persist in such craziness.

Babysitters (Or Yes, You Can Leave Melissa for a While—And Melissa Needs Some Time Away from You)

You feel guilty, nervous, you'll never be able to enjoy yourself. *Garbage!* You've *got* to get out, Mr. and Ms. Parents of a sugar baby. One of the things we often talk about at JDF meetings is the horrendous strain that diabetes can create in a marriage, and too much togetherness with Melissa will do it every time. You absolutely need time to retrench, recoup your capacity for silliness or romance or solitude. Babysitters are the solution, and they can be grandparents, mature teenagers, or that nice, cool retired lady or man down the block. The key word is "cool." You can't leave anyone with your little one who is more apt to lose her cool than you are. Very often a sensible teenager will do far better than devoted but very Noivous Grandmother. One couple said this at a meeting: "For the first year we didn't leave his side to go out—anywhere. One day, we finally left him for two hours with Tom's aunt and we called four times in those two hours. When we got back she told us, 'You're trying to be beta cells instead of parents.' It was true."

1. If your worst fear is that your child will have an insulin reaction with a sitter who can't handle it, make sure you choose a sitter who is comfortable with a crash course on diabetes and how to handle emergencies. Love is not enough. If one set of grandparents thinks injections are a piece of cake and the other set simply cannot do it, no matter how hard they try or love the child, don't force the issue—let them be. Sleep-over dates at Grandma's will have to be limited to the grandma who can cope with emergency. But all grandparents, copers or not, should be very much included in a child's life, needless to say. Understand that some people may be emotionally willing to deal with injections but psychologically unable to do it.

2. A good way to handle the crash course is to "role-play" an emergency with your potential sitter after you've given her instructions. Set up the situation—

Okay, Melissa doesn't seem to respond; she's cold and clammy and pale and staring but not talking. What do you do? Then you go through each step, acting out the getting of the sugar, the glucagon, the calling of the doctor, etc. You'd be surprised—it's much easier to handle an emergency if you've walked through the steps.

And expect to take time to train a babysitter. One father says: "It took two and a half months to train my nineteen-year-old sister until she and we felt comfortable leaving her with Sharon. First we worked on the shots, then the emergency situations, and slowly, we brought her along. Up until then, we'd been using registered nurses as sitters; it cost us a fortune to go to a movie."

3. Always leave a phone number where you can be reached or where a good, capable friend can be reached. The phone number of a parent with a diabetic child is a wonderful number to leave because that parent will know what to do in most emergencies. Your local JDF chapter can supply you with that. Besides phone numbers, leave a general idea of where you'll be if you're not at someone's house. You can be paged at the A&P, the movies, almost anywhere.

4. ALWAYS leave the doctor's telephone number and the number of the emergency ambulance of your local hospital.

5. Always have fresh orange juice in the refrigerator . . . ready to use, *not* in frozen cans. Be sure to leave your sugar sources and glucagon within easy, visible reach. Leave detailed instructions about foods to feed and snacks that are available. Leave proper *times* of feeding available.

6. Be sure *to spell out* the simplest of instructions: you'd be surprised to find how many people don't understand the seriousness of saying "No sweets" ("Oh, just this one Tootsie Roll won't hurt").

7. The most wonderful and reassuring kind of babysitting system is one that many JDF parents have set up. Either they take turns sitting with each other's children, with their own in a spare room, or one set of parents is elected to be "on call" in their own home should an emergency arise with a babysitter. It's a great feeling to leave your child with a babysitter knowing that there are experienced parents within a block or a phone call away, should your sitter need help.

Start out small, with sitters, an hour or so at first, then a whole evening. Very soon, believe it or not, you'll even be able to take a vacation alone with your husband (or lover, whichever the case may be). You'll all survive . . . honest!

The Sick Days

They happen—and they're no reason for unnecessary alarm. If you've been sent on a fear trip by a foolish doctor (they're around) or an uninformed relative who tells you that it's *very* dangerous for children with diabetes to get sick, get off that crummy roller coaster right now! It's true that you have two jobs instead of one: not only do you have to get that child better but you also have to make sure that his/her diabetes stays in reasonable control. Of course, you can do it; but living in fear of infection it can be both destructive and scary. The properly informed parents of a little one with diabetes should operate with the quiet knowledge that most childhood illnesses are no big deal.

Sometimes it's difficult to tell if your baby is sick or just plain cranky. If he/she didn't have diabetes, it wouldn't be essential to guess the correct reasons for unhappiness. Having a baby with diabetes, though, requires you to be more than a good guesser. You have to be a terrific tester. Thank goodness for blood tests and also urine tests! The former lets you know right away if the blood sugar high. If it is, and the baby has other identifying signs of illness (red throat, swollen glands, maybe funny little spots signifying measles, etc.), you can assume some kind of infection. The stress of illness almost invariably raises blood sugar, you see. If a urine test shows signs of ketones, that, *along with* high blood sugar, indicates a need for more insulin—right away. Make sure you find out from your doctor just what amount to give.

Things to remember on sick days

1. *Give That Shot!* Your cute, sweet little kid is just too weak for the insulin shot, and anyway he's hardly eating so he probably can do without it? *Wrong!* If the kid's not too sick to breathe, he's not too sick for his insulin shot. Because illness tends to cause a rise in blood sugar, he needs at least his usual dosage and maybe even more (of the regular or fast-acting insulin) to compensate for the higher sugar. Your goal is not only to get him better but to prevent acidosis from setting in. How much extra insulin? Dr. George P. Kozak—who is head of the Department of Endocrinology at New England Deaconess Hospital in Brookline, Mass., and also works at the Joslin Clinic—says that *if* ketones are present with a rise in blood sugar, 20 percent of the usual daily dose added on as a supplement of insulin is a safe place to start. And always check with your doctor if the ketones and high blood sugar persist after several supplements.

During any illness, the doctor-parent partnership should be in effect. Don't hesitate to call and re-call the doctor to make sure the insulin dosage is correct. Treatment of diabetes should consist of the doctor being the adviser and prescriber and the parent the effector of the prescribed treatment.

2. *Give That Hug!* No kidding. This is a time for more hugs and

tender loving care. Research has shown that touching reduces stress and that has not only a psychological effect on your baby. Dr. Dolores Krieger of the Mount Sinai Hospital in New York, an expert on "therapeutic touch," has proven conclusively that the power of touch is massive and wonderful for its curative value. If stress can raise the blood sugar of a baby with diabetes, hugs and kisses and stroking, which soothe stress, are better than Mother's chicken soup.

3. If you have given extra insulin to the toddler, it's a good idea to check his sugar during the night. If his illness is getting better, he may now have a *low* blood sugar because of the extra insulin and may need a snack or some sugar.

4. Hotline: you need one to your doctor, and hotlines work at night, too. Make sure you have his home phone number so you can be in contact in non-office hours and don't hesitate to call at 3:00 A.M. if you really need to. Don't hesitate, also, to change doctors if you sense an irritation with these extra ungodly-hour calls. If he/she agrees to treat a child with diabetes, that goes with the territory.

5. Nausea and vomiting are common in childhood illnesses and they're crummy for diabetes control. You *must* control the vomiting. See the section on "The Emergencies" (pp. 24–33) to find out how.

6. Beware of medication that is not prescribed by a thoroughly knowledgeable doctor. Many medicines (cough medicines are the worst offenders) contain sugar. When your baby's small body is producing even more sugar because of her illness, she certainly doesn't need a sugar kick in her cough elixir. There are sugar-free cough medicines; they include Cidicol, Diametapp Elixir, and Tussar S.F. Other medications may interact poorly with insulin (cortisone and Dilantin, for instance), *so always check with a doctor who is expert at diabetes care*, even if another doctor prescribed the medication. (Some sugar-free medicines can also affect diabetes.)

7. Exercise can aggravate illness, so cancel your child's calisthenics for the duration of the illness.

8. Drinking is especially important. If your baby just won't eat solids, try small sips of milk, sweetened fruit juices, ginger ale or Coke, soup. Salty broth is great if there's a lot of vomiting or fever because it replaces lost minerals. Try easy-to-digest foods now like yogurt, ice cream, oatmeal, crackers, cottage cheese, eggs, toast—in small amounts, not big meals.

9. For diarrhea: try Kaopectate. Ask your doctor about an intramuscular injection of Compazine or Tigan.

And so, on to the next stage, the Sugar Kids. When your very young child develops and acquires that miracle of all miracles, speech, she'll be able to help you immensely. One of the most frustrating things about having a baby with diabetes is that you can't tell how she feels before verbal communication is established. As the years pass and her capacity for self-regulation grows, diabetes gets a lot easier to handle. If there is any one bit of advice to pass down that is true for every single family of a child with juvenile diabetes it's this: reach out to other families with the same problems and the same victories. Rap sessions with others give you new techniques to try, new outlooks to consider. Even if you are a family that has never sought help from anyone else before, do it now. You can't imagine how good it will feel.

2 SUGAR KIDS

Let's start with a twelve-year-old, first.

The scene is a creative writing class in a Beverly Hills elementary school and the assignment has sparked no more than mild interest in the sun-jaded eleven- and twelve-year-olds of Movie City. The teacher is working on the technique called *Process:* the ability to clearly explain how something works, step by step. Each kid is to get up in front of the class and teach his peers to do something. So far the class has "learned" how to tie a shoelace, write a report, and make an ice-cream soda, step by stultifying step. The class is yawning audibly. So is the teacher. She's secretly thinking, one more shoelace, one more seltzer bottle, and she'll retire.

Then, it's Leslie's turn.

"Some of you know, and some of you don't, that I have diabetes," she says, a little nervously. "I'm going to teach you how to make a blood test for sugar."

Twenty-three kids perk up visibly. Blood? Yeccch. It has great possibilities . . .

Then Leslie, carefully, graphically went through the routine with which she'd become a pro by this time, having been diagnosed as diabetic at seven. First she explained what diabetes is. Then she explained what blood sugar is and why it was important to keep track of it. And then she swabbed her finger with alcohol, pricked it, and dropped the specimen on a test strip. The kids watched with bated breath. What color would it turn? Cream? Good. Purple? Oh, no . . . It was moss green, 25 mg. of sugar, not so bad, said Leslie. She put the strip into a reflectance meter which gave her a digital reading and it turned out she had less sugar than she thought.

You could hear a pin drop. Then, questions, questions, a million questions. The kids were fascinated. Leslie was prepared with the answers because no one knew more about her own diabetes than she did. "But I thought it was curable with insulin. . . ?"

"Is that why you're always good for a Lifesaver?"

"Is it catching?"

She was the star of the class, a person who was able to deal with self-disclosure—to share parts of her true self and feelings. But make no mistake. This shining, delightful, interesting child had gone through some rocky times to get to the point where she was able to discuss diabetes so competently. And she had some difficult times ahead, as the handling of the disease changed its implications at various stages of her life—college, marriage, pregnancy. But, all in all, this twelve-year-old had it made. She was in control of her life as well as her diabetes. With the help of her family, doctors, and now, with the understanding of her friends, she was not a diabetic youngster but a youngster who had diabetes—along with a lot of *terrific* things in her life. Some choose not to share themselves, but Leslie wanted her peers to know. Besides, it made for a great answer to the assignment.

Nine kids lined up to have their own blood sugar tested.

As our little ones are preparing to start the great adventure of school, we parents are nothing less than wrecks. I could have said we are concerned, we are edgy, we have doubts—but that really wouldn't do. What we are is unmitigated, sometimes hair-pulling sometimes nail-biting *wrecks.* Will he have an insulin reaction and lie there unconscious before someone notices him? Will he forget to eat his snack? Will the kids sense something "different" about him and shun him? Will he be able to manage without me?

The answer to that last question is, Yes. He will.

But in certain ways he *is* different from the others. Whoever tries to tell you otherwise is talking nonsense—and you both know it! Diabetes *can* be life-threatening if insulin is not taken and if diet and activity are not carefully monitored. What's more, although your child doesn't have to walk around with a scarlet D on his chest, it is essential that many people know about his disease and how to help him if the need arises. No question about it, there are differences.

Yet the good news is that the differences are manageable and that your child with diabetes can do absolutely everything the other kids can do, including playing, taking tests, making friends, exploring, going to parties—everything. He can even eat sweets on special occasions so he won't feel left out (more on that later).

The bad news is that he has to *prepare* for the things he chooses to do ... and you have to help him assume that responsibility, little by little. This means that although diabetes doesn't have to be uppermost in his or your mind every day, it does have to be in there, somewhere, almost all the time. It's not too early to start developing a lifetime habit of thoughtfulness, of awareness of what you and he need to do now and what you'll need to do in two hours to keep this disease in control. After a while, the whole routine comes pretty naturally.

The single most important thing at this and at future ages is that *you be absolutely truthful about this disease with your child.* There's no more reason why a veil of secrecy, fear, and shame should hover around the management of diabetes than about the management of a broken leg. The goal is for you eventually to step out of the centerstage and allow the disease to belong to your child—as it does. Eventually, he will make the decisions about the way he wants to live with it, and that should happen gradually, starting now. If he does not know the truth about what to expect and what not to expect, if he is handed sugar-coated platitudes, then he cannot be expected to do a good job.

The reason you ought to always tell your child the truth is because the truth about diabetes contains much optimism and positive thought. Although the person who said to you when you first found out, "Thank God it's only diabetes!" (everyone has had someone say that to them) was a jerk because diabetes is no picnic, it's also not the most terrible. You can grow up with diabetes and you can grow old with diabetes, if you're informed and alert.

As parents with children in school, our goals should be:

• to protect our young children without being overprotective
• to keep close tabs on them and, at the same time, start to let go
• to prepare our children for self-responsibility and self-care.

An easy, mellow, relaxed atmosphere rather than a strict, no-yield home helps more than you would imagine. It ain't easy, as the sage said, but it *can* be done. Here's how many of us have handled it . . .

KINDERGARTEN TIME

You may have lived with diabetes for some time now; as a result, you've learned to make many adjustments and to deal beautifully with new situations as they crop up. You've got a big adjustment coming up this year, if your child is about to start school, because in your heart of hearts you think that you alone are absolutely indispensable to Jill's well-being. Who else would be able to catch her special signals of shockiness that even she cannot yet recognize? Well, lots of people will be able to do just that, with your help. Here are some guidelines put together from parents who have been through it.

The First Step: Educating the Educators

Before school begins, make an appointment to see *in person* every adult who will have anything to do with your child's day. That includes Jill's

- regular teacher
- school nurse
- principal
- any specialty teachers (sports, arts and crafts, etc.).

Do it very soon before the beginning of school, rather than a month before, so that the information will be fresh in their consciousnesses. You can meet with them together so that the management of Jill's diabetes will be a joint effort and no surprise to anyone. What do you tell them? Order copies of the booklet *What You Should Know About the Student with Diabetes,* put out by the Juvenile Diabetes Foundation, and give one to each teacher.

Among the facts that should be presented at your meeting are (1) *a very short explanation of what diabetes is* (don't take it for granted that even the school nurse knows); and (2) *what happens* and *what to look for should an insulin reaction set in.* It's also important to tell them that your child will have to eat a mid-morning and mid-afternoon snack, *on time.* Stress that if the snack is not eaten on time in the morning, Jill may have a low blood sugar reaction before lunch. If the mid-afternoon snack is missed, it could spell trouble on the way home. Although hypoglycemia is what the school will be most concerned with, you might want to give them the symptoms of high blood sugar (hyperglycemia), which is not of too much concern to the school officials because it comes on so slowly.

Every adult who teaches your child should be prepared with a supply of sugar in the form of candy or sweetened juice. The school nurse should be provided with

- doctor's telephone numbers
- parent's telephone numbers
- a supply of crackers, cheese (the squirt kind that keeps without re-frigeration), juice, and paper cups

It's so important to impress on the adults who will teach your child that she not be singled out as an "invalid." She can do everything, *if* her disease is in control. Encourage Jill's teacher to call you if she has any questions, and keep her posted on the things that may directly affect Jill's day. Since illness and emotional stress can make blood sugar rise, the teacher should be notified if you think Jill has a cold coming on, if Jill's sister was rotten to her in the morning, which *could* cause a rise in sugar, if Jill is upset about *anything*. Tell the teacher what to do about throwing up should Jill feel nauseous. Jill should keep a snack in her desk and the teacher should have one on hand also, for emergencies. And finally, you should follow up this initial process of education with regular school conferences, throughout the year, to answer and ask questions of each other.

What Next?—A Medley of Problems That Can Pop Up

You've been very used to making your own schedules for Jill. Now you will have to follow a whole lot of other people's schedules. This is where both you and your child begin to learn flexibility.

Buses If your child will go on a bus ride to get to school, find out the schedule so you can plan breakfast times. There's to be no dashing out the door with a bite of waffle. She *must* eat before school, so allow time for nervousness, for "not being hungry," for insulin shots, for dressing, so that you can meet that bus without getting everyone nutso. Figure on at least a half an hour for breakfast.

Scheduling You're used to giving Jill lunch at noon, but she's been scheduled to an afternoon kindergarten session. She'll have to eat lunch at eleven so she can get to school on time. If it means a longer period of time without food in the early afternoon (with a resulting blood sugar drop), Jill will have to have a larger snack at three o'clock than usual.

Changes in Insulin You may not only have to manipulate the eating but make some changes in her insulin dosage. Although Jill's been taking more regular than NPH or Lente, you may have to add more longer-lasting insulin now, so that she will be covered for the longer day if she has a school trip or something like that. If the school schedule for any reason might delay her lunch, you'll have to make sure she either has a snack to eat to compensate or a reduction in her regular insulin shot in the morning. In the spring and summertime, the kindergarten children will be playing out-side, probably, and the spurt of activity will use up more carbohydrates.

Think ahead, question the teacher as to her plans for the week, if possible, and manipulate the food and insulin requirements accordingly, after consulting with your doctor.

Gym Time If this falls right before lunch, a larger morning snack might be required.

Snack Time If Jill needs to eat her snack at a time when no one else is snacking, it might cause problems. Jill's peers might not think so kindly about a kid who gets to eat crackers and they get to eat nothing . . . and it doesn't help to explain very much, either. Most kids couldn't care less if Jill was pregnant, had the plague, or anything else. "It's not fair," would be the reaction, rest assured.

A little foresight can handle this. If she feels funny leaving the class each day to eat her snack, perhaps the teacher can arrange a daily "job" for her that will take her out of the classroom—say the bringing of attendance cards to the office or the collection of the teacher's mail from the office. Since many other kids have daily "jobs," this is an easy out and a way for Jill to eat that snack. It's wise to leave it up to her whether to tell or not to tell her classmates about her diabetes, let alone the snack. One mother says that her child's jewel of a teacher arranged for the whole class to snack when her son was scheduled to eat, and then that teacher sat with her son each day to make sure he *finished* his snack. That's dedication—also self-preservation.

Glucagon Permission? Some states allow a school nurse to give a glucagon shot, although most do not. Check to see what the rules in your state are.

Shocky Provisions Even if the teacher and the nurse are prepared with sugar sources and quick energy supplies for Jill, she should never leave the house without some easy-to-carry candy for emergencies and a small amount of quick energy food, like raisins or an orange. The candy is for when she's feeling a reaction coming on (naturally, you have to be able to trust her that she'll save it for just this time) and the quick energy food is to be used before unexpected gym class, recess, or other carbohydrate-expending activity. Tell her to check with her teacher before she eats it, just to make sure there's some adult supervision involved. The extra food is also good to have for *after* insulin reaction has been treated with sugar.

In the end, your child will learn instinctively to tell when she has too much or too little sugar in her system (and most kids do learn that). Then she also has to be able to find the strength to act on her knowledge. If a substitute teacher tells her she can't leave the room when she *knows* she has to go visit the nurse for a snack, she must learn that she has to get up and leave. She has to be prepared to question teachers, question any authority who tells her she can't do a thing that she knows she *must* do for her own health. It's a hard thing to learn—no doubt about it. Grown-ups who say they know what's best look awfully big to an eleven-year-old, let alone a seven-year-old. But once she's started to develop the courage of her convictions, with your help and advice, your Jill will learn to be a self-asserting, absolutely fine person . . . and probably way ahead of a "normal" kid who doesn't have these early lessons in conviction and self-assurance.

A QUESTION OF ATTITUDE

No cutesy title, here. This is serious stuff. We're talking about the attitude of the person who has diabetes, and her family's attitude as well. It counts as much as keeping blood sugar down—and that's no exaggeration.

If your child thinks diabetes will destroy her life, it probably will. If she thinks it's a bummer, sure, but one she can handle, we can guarantee that her life will be as joyful and productive as if she didn't have the bummer.

In many magazines and books, even in this book, you've read that the disease is your child's disease, not yours. You've read that the responsibility for the disease should be given over to her. Well, up to a point, that advice is solid.

Dr. Fredda Ginsberg-Fellner, director of the Division of Pediatric Endocrinology and Metabolism at the Mount Sinai School of Medicine in New York, maintains that brand-new evidence in the form of psychologic studies indicates that the disease, if handled properly, is a family's disease, after all, not just one person's responsibility. "Support systems are vital," she stresses. "Any family that says, 'Hey, we're not going to stop having all this good junk food around just because of her,' is looking for disaster." That kind of attitude is bound to make a child with diabetes feel depressed and isolated. To say, "It's *his* problem," will sure as shooting give everyone else a problem. It's important for a child with diabetes to assume responsibility, of course, but it's equally important for him to know that everyone else in his life is pulling for him and cheering him on, even if this involves certain limited deprivations for the rest of the family.

Having a good attitude means keeping your adult anxiety level low. If you set *reasonable* goals for your child's testing, dieting, exercise, you can avoid most of the no-win confrontations that occur between parents and kids who don't easily accept yokes of blame, guilt, defensiveness, and anger.

Attitude means, even if it sounds cruel, not being a bleeding heart. Feeling sorry for the kid who has diabetes doesn't help one bit. Sure, all the things she has to do are not pleasant, but they're not hell on wheels either, and aching for your kid tears down her self-image and adds little to her sense of competence. That does not mean no hugs and sympathy: on the contrary, it means *more* hugs and less pity, nagging, or constant reminding. No school absences should ever be due to diabetes: if your attitude says that diabetes is not "sickly," your child's attitude will follow suit. If your child feels shocky in the morning and says she doesn't want to go to school because the spelling test will surely bring it on again—don't buy it.

There's an ugly word that has sprung up in our diabetes vocabulary, and that word is "compliance." By compliance, the doctors mean that a kid should be willing to stick to a routine that will keep his diabetes in control. But the definition of compliance is "yielding to a wish or demand: a disposition to yield to others." How would you like to do all that yielding to others? I goes against the grain of human nature to be so damn compliant.

In contrast, if a child learns gradually that certain acts have certain consequences, he'll be yielding to his *own* head, which tells him what feels good. There is no better authority. If he skips his insulin, feels crummy afterwards, and has acetones in his urine, that's a much stronger reason to take his insulin than because his mother and doctor require compliance. There should be very little not wanting to go to school because of diabetes if a young person understands that his own actions are the ones that bring about the consequences, good or bad.

Attitude also means not placing value judgments on the state of your child's physical self. For years, we've been saying that our children's urine tests were either "bad" or "good." When the tests showed sugar, they were "bad"—and, as a result, the hidden message was that the kid was also bad. The converse was true: "good" tests meant a good kid. No wonder so many of the kids were faking results, drinking gallons of water to change urine sugar, lying to their doctors. Anybody would do that. Today we know that often blood sugar has nothing to do with how "good" the kid's been, because hormonal changes, stress, any number of extraneous things can make a "bad" result into a "good" one, and vice versa.

Okay: end of lecture. Just know that attitude moves mountains. If you and your child fully expect life to be uncomplicated and routine, with no sharp peaks and valleys *due to diabetes,* it no doubt will be. Attitude doesn't come naturally; you have to work on it. But, no kidding, even if you're a wild, nervous Crazy—you can change. You owe it to your kid to try.

Happy Birthday!

What do you tell an eight-year-old who is going to his best friend's birthday party? Do you tell him that he can't have any birthday cake and he can't have any ice cream? If you do, you're likely to be thought of in a less than loving light.

He *can* have some treats, you know. Although heaven would consist of junk food every day for some people, children with diabetes cannot party every day. But once in a while? Sure. The goal is to allow your little one to feel as normal as possible, to meld in with the others, as well as to develop leadership capability. And melding often *demands* birthday cake when you're eight. So you teach him to take the icing off. And you teach him to have only a small portion of ice cream. You plan ahead, as we suggested earlier, and you try to compensate for the treat you know is coming. You give a little extra insulin in his morning injection. Perhaps you speak to his friend's mother and ask her to provide artificially sweetened ice cream, Jello, lemonade, or soda for your child, without making it obvious that she's doing so.

As he gets older, he'll have to surely learn to limit his sugar intake by himself: you can't ask his friend's mother do so when he's eighteen without incurring funny looks. But a rare birthday treat will not be the end of the world. If it happens too often, though, and you compensate with extra insulin and less food regularly, his diabetes control will be shot to heck and the yo-yo syndrome it often produces (low to high to low to high, etc., blood sugar) can have unfortunate consequences in the future. The trick is to avoid rigidity in everything, even diet. Forbidden fruit has a way of looking irresistibly attractive; allowing it once in a while takes the overpowering appeal away.

Oi Vey, It's Halloween Again!

Of all the holidays that stand for fun to most families, Halloween most strikes fear into the hearts of parents who have children with diabetes. It's not fear of poisoned candy but fear of sugar that's a problem to these parents. It really is a pain, but it must be dealt with. First thing you can do (and you can only do this when your kid is very young, not apt to wander away from the block) is to alert your immediate neighbors where your child will be visiting to provide apples, diet candies, nuts, dried raisins, popcorn, dried fruits, and other acceptable Halloween treats.

The minute little Jason is allowed to stray from the neighborly womb, he's got to be instructed carefully. Number one: he must learn that he *may not* eat anything while out on the trail. That's pretty easy to do because most of the kids are so busy collecting, they have no time for sampling. When he gets home, try these strategies.

The Substitution Ploy   It's sneaky, but it works when they're little. Just have some identical "loot bags" filled and ready with good stuff to be surreptitiously switched with the bad stuff loot bag. Good stuff can be raisins, apples, raw carrot curls.

The Barter Ploy   Your child will look forward, after a while, to the bartering game. It works like this: you "trade" twenty-five boxes of candy for twenty-five boxes of raisins. Or you trade a box of dietetic candies for a Hershey bar. Or you trade a late night stay-up for a package of licorice in the offending bag. Either way, knowing that a Halloween present is the reward for giving up the candy makes Halloween far less frustrating for your child.

The Save for Later Ploy   You divide the loot up into the stuff that's okay to eat now and the stuff that's to be saved for when the child is feeling shocky. Then the offending Chunky bars and Good 'n Plenty's can be stored in a closet for those days when your child is experiencing mild insulin reactions. We must admit, there's a danger in this one: youngsters desperate to eat the candy may fabricate a "shocky" reaction when there is none, or may even cut down on a scheduled snack to create a shocky feeling. You know your own child, and that should be the deciding factor on what ploy to use. One thing is sure: Halloween candy may *not* be gobbled up "just this once." It would be a disastrous precedent, let alone a disastrous blood sugar reading. Gentle firmness should rule the day. If you are wishy-washy or vacillating in your desire to make Jason happy, he'll sense your indecision in a moment. A good dietary routine should never—well, hardly ever—be invaded ruthlessly. (Rare birthday party treats are not ruthless invasions.)

SHOULD KAREN GO TO CAMP?

Of course, Karen can go to camp, in case you've been wondering. In fact, with the proper preparation, away-from-home situations like camp not only include your child in the mainstream of life but they teach her how to care for herself at an early age . . . a wonderful bonus! The other day, we met a child of twelve who had never been away from her mother's side, let alone given herself her own shots. She's been away from her father's side, all right, because her parents were divorced. Who could live with a wife who made diabetes management her raison d'être, who refused to allow her child to claim her own disease? That kind of situation should never be allowed and a built-in weaning away can happen at camp.

How old should your child be? Depends upon the kid, of course, but most camps begin accepting campers at the age of six; programs usually continue until they're fifteen and then they can be counselors-in-training. The only decision is—do you send your child to a special camp for diabetic youngsters or to a regular camp with understanding and knowledgeable personnel?

Many of us at the Juvenile Diabetes Foundation tend to go with the regular camps precisely because we feel that we can't isolate our kids from the "norm" throughout their lives, nor do we wish to. There are, thank goodness, no special colleges for young adults with diabetes, nor are there any special offices, marriage plans, or vacation spots. Still, there are certain advantages to special camps. For the newly diagnosed diabetic child who needs help learning the new language and confusing rules of diabetes, being in a place where everyone speaks the same language is a great boon. For the child who contracted diabetes as a baby and never really learned a proper self-care routine, a special camp is very helpful. For the child whose parents are unspeakably overprotective, making her feel like a fragile, delicate work of art that can't do anything, being in a place where all the children with diabetes run and jump and play as hard as they possibly can is quite a revelation and quite a comfort. And finally, for the child who *uses* her diabetes at home to get special privileges from family and friends, being in a place where everybody has the same illness makes the illness no big deal and not good for special attention. For these kids, we agree, a special camp seems like a good idea.

Again, the name of the game is choice. Look into regular camps, check into the camps for children who have diabetes, then make an informed choice. The Juvenile Diabetes Foundation can send you a complete list of camps for diabetic children. Financial assistance is generally available if you need it.

Naturally, it goes without saying that if you opt for the regular camp, you'll check the whole thing out with the camp directors (before you tell your child) first. Many directors refuse to accept the responsibility of a child with diabetes, and JDF parents tell us they've been flatly refused, even hung up on, when telephoning for information in such camps whose directors are uninformed, nervous, nasty, or just plain stupid.

One of the big bonuses of summer camp for your child is that it gives *you* a little breather from the day-to-day management—no small present. Your relationships with your spouse and other children in the family who don't have diabetes can get a shot in the arm, not of insulin but of confidence and caring. When a diabetic child is getting all the attention, or most of it, anyway, feelings of deprivation are common among the others. There's nothing like a month or so of time alone with parents to rejuvenate bruised feelings. The diabetic child gets a new support system to help him realize he can live without his parents, and the others in the family get some spotlights of their own.

So, whatever you decide about types of camp, unless your child would be psychologically devastated by separation, there's nothing better for everyone concerned than camp. The chance for a child with diabetes to burst free from overprotective or even very cool parents is a truly liberating experience. Hooray for the White Team!

In a Nutshell . . . Pros and Cons of Special Camps

PROS	CONS
There's a well-protected environment of fellow diabetics and very well trained personnel, many of whom have diabetes themselves.	It *is* a form of isolation from the real world, no matter how you look at it.
Programs of urine and blood testing, nutritional advice, and emotional succor geared especially to the child with diabetes are often available.	There's no reason why a kid can't do everything in a regular camp, *if* the adults in charge and his/her immediate peers are well educated to the needs of diabetes.
The child often finds relief and companionship with others who have the same problems. This can be comforting.	Special camps focus attention on the illness sometimes more than on the whole kid.
There are no after-nap cookies and malted milk snacks for the skinny kids—and for the kids with diabetes to steel themselves against.	Most special camps have only two-week sessions. Parents *and* kids could often use a longer vacation from each other.
Special camps are particularly good for newly diagnosed diabetics, who may need help in learning confusing new routines.	
They reinforce the diabetic self-care regimen for those who forgot or never learned properly.	
They remove any excuses for special attention solely because of the disease.	

SPORTS . . . YES, HE CAN PLAY BALL

—Or swim, or jog, or chase a tennis ball around. Having diabetes does not preclude a youngster from vigorous sports activity. When his diabetes is under control, he can be the star of the baseball team (if he can hit, that is). Naturally, he's got to still keep taking insulin, despite the form of a popular myth which says that if you exercise, you can stop insulin (which incidentally is absolutely untrue). The reason for the myth is this: Exercise, long called the invisible insulin, in a way does the same thing as insulin—it causes the body to use up sugar. But what it does is make less insulin necessary, not cut out the need for it altogether. So it's important for a sports-addicted youngster to keep taking his insulin and eating properly.

Being active in sports is a super way to keep weight down and to increase blood circulation, both important to the child with diabetes. Many professional athletes are diabetics who have used sports to make them "healthy diabetics"; baseball star Ron Santo and tennis pro Billy Talbert are examples, to name just two.

One thing to look out for when your child is a serious sports partici-pant is low blood sugar, which comes when heavy exercise uses up sugar and there's still too much insulin working in the body. You can handle this in one of two ways; either have her snack quite a bit more before an athletic event, or eat only a little more and take less insulin the day of such an event. If your child seems to get about the same amount of sports activity every day, then a protein snack of milk, cheese, or meat before running the race (or whatever) will help prevent a blood sugar drop. If you know that her exercise will be sporadic and that there's a big swim event, say, one day a week, perhaps your doctor will suggest an insulin adjustment for those special days.

Dr. Alicia Schiffrin, pediatric endocrinologist with Montreal Chil-dren's Hospital, says that exercise will generally decrease insulin needs but not in all children. It is necessary to play it by ear, with each child, she advises, watching individual requirements and decreasing insulin as the patient's blood sugar changes—if it does—with activity. Entertainment star and tennis pro Dan Rowan lowers his insulin before a tournament, but hockey pro Bobby Clarke prefers to fool with the amount of food he takes in rather than tampering with the insulin. It all depends on your child's schedule, physical condition, and his doctor's advice. For young kids, it's often more advisable to change the food rather than the insulin intake, because if the game is called due to poor weather, or the coach decides not to play him the day he expected to star in all four quarters, he's not locked into a lesser insulin dose. You can always grab a snack right *before* you have to jump into the game, but you can't be quite so flexible with insulin shots.

Another thing to consider in connection with heavy exercise is blood pressure. Dr. Fredda Ginsberg-Fellner says: "If I had a young child with an elevated blood pressure or even a question of that, I'd certainly do a stress test on that child to see if heavy exercise will make that pressure rise. Although this is a problem mostly with people who have had diabetes for ten years or over, it *can* apply to young children also."

It's necessary *always* to be prepared with a snack in case there is an insulin reaction. Your youngster must clearly understand that if he/she feels shocky during the meet, diabetes comes first, and not the point. In other words, there's to be no waiting till the inning's over to take that needed sugar fix: time-outs are a kid's best friend. If your youngster's sports activities take him to places like a mountain trail or a ski slope where there's no handy candy machine, he must be doubly prepared with his own food: His life depends on it.

Okay, so you know that sports are terrific for the youngster with diabetes. What you may not know is that, very often, children tend to blame their disease for failures of any sort. If your daughter says she didn't make the swim team because of her diabetes, sit down and talk about it. It's skill that's the name of the game in competition and diabetes *never* has anything to do with that. It's always unfortunate to see anyone cop out with an excuse of diabetes when it's tough to face things realistically. If you go along with a kid who thinks of himself as an invalid, chances are he will become one.

NOTE: Children with diabetes should *never* partake in sports alone. The buddy system saves lives. If his/her sport is a rather solitary activity by nature, like hiking, mountain climbing, jogging, surfing, snorkeling, cycling, boating, or exploring caves, always be sure that he tells someone nearby that he is a diabetic . . . and checks in with that person fairly regularly.

But you still don't love him out there playing football no matter what you read in this book!

Naturally, you don't. You'd be lying through your teeth if you said that as a parent of a child with diabetes, you don't have many more anxieties about sports than a parent of a child without the disease. You have not only the major broken leg to worry about, but the small cut, infection, bruise stuff, because nothing can be lightly sloughed off in this disease. You worry about blistering, healing, and shockiness while the other kids' parents are just worried about his making the goal.

Okay, so you worry. The trick is to keep most of it to yourself, even if you're absolutely certain that it's your worrying alone that's kept your child reasonably whole up until now. One mother we know puts it this way: "I used to speak to coaches behind his back, asking them to watch out for signs of shockiness. I used to call him twelve times a night when he played away from home and slept at another kid's house. I used to follow him around from game to game, always ready with the orange juice. It's a miracle he didn't either kill me or run away from home."

It *is* destructive to try to pad your child against all possible happenings. That's a sure way for a person to grow up an emotional cripple. This is not to say you have to relinquish all authority completely. On the contrary, even if your child is ashamed to carry the juice himself or look like a coach's pet because he gets special snacking privileges, be tough and ignore those particular sensibilities. He carries the juice, he eats the snacks, or he doesn't play the game. Simple and firm as that.

It may happen that you run into a doctor who thinks sports are not important for a diabetic youngster and advises against them in the name of caution. My advice to you is, get another doctor. There's controversy about the benefits of exercise as there is in most other matters pertaining to the management of diabetes, but the newest and best information tells us that activity is terrific for a young child with diabetes—or for anyone with diabetes, for that matter. The diabetic child should not be restricted in any way as far as his physical activity is concerned. On the contrary, he or she must be encouraged to participate in all manner of sports and athletics. Adequate physical exercise is helpful not only in terms of psychological implications but because insufficient exercise is one of the factors that raises blood sugar levels and alters insulin requirements.

It's also possible that you run into a doctor who is lukewarm about sports because he himself has never put sneaker to foot. The thing to do is to educate yourself by doing as much reading as possible, as much asking of questions as possible, and then make an informed decision about sports for your child. Encourage him to go out for exercise. He may never become a Catfish Hunter (another famous athlete with diabetes), but he should not be stopped from trying.

One last word on sports activity: Suppose you're all in favor of it, your doctor is also, your child is raring to go for Little League—and the Little League coach nixes the whole thing because he thinks

- diabetes is catching
- diabetics are prone to die while catching fly balls
- he just doesn't want the responsibility.

Nothing left but to educate the coach and/or whoever has the responsibility for deciding who shall play and who shall not. Make it a point to have your doctor write a longish note spelling out your child's ability to participate. Make an appointment to share your knowledge with uninformed authorities. Make it a point also to tell the coach, as you're educating him, that he's not to single out your child even to give him special privileges because of his disease. That would defeat the whole purpose of honest participation in the game.

TRAVEL: YOU DO IT WITH DIABETES, NOT FROM DIABETES

You're dying to go to Pennsylvania, but how can you leave home, your medicine chest, your doctor, with a child who has diabetes? You're pining for Paris, but going out of the country is unthinkable? Think again . . . and start packing! There's no reason on earth why you can't travel anywhere, which includes the town next door as well as the country next door. The operative words are PREPARE and LISTS. Your mother always told you to make lists, and boy, was she right when it comes to being on the move with a chronic disease. If you are ready for any emergency, you can relax and rest assured that nine times out of ten, there won't be one.

On a plane, boat, or in a car, always assume the worst will happen:

- gridlock for seven hours
- bad weather, which keeps you circling the airport for three hours
- mind-boggling traffic
- pirates.

Before You Go

Never go anywhere without a security blanket of a small suitcase packed with:

- food: packaged cheese crackers, containers of juice, Coke, fruit
- quick sugar sources like cake gels, honey, a supply of glucagon
- insulin and extra syringes: take enough to last the whole trip, and then a few extra. Never send insulin through the luggage system, which eats suitcases. Carry it with you as personal hand luggage (airport X-rays won't hurt it).

It's possible you will go to a place where the insulin you use (U-100) is not available and where you may have to take U-40 or U-80 strength. Write to the manufacturer of the insulin you use to ask about its availability in the places you're going to, and ask, also, how to adapt your dosage to U-40 or U-80 strengths.* The addresses of the manufacturers follow:

Eli Lilly & Company
Medical Dept.
307 East McCarty St.
Indianapolis, Ind. 46285

Squibb-Novo Inc.
120 Alexander St.
Princeton, N. J. 08540

Nordisk
6500 Rock Spring Drive
Bethesda, Md. 20817

---

*See also the chart on human insulin in "III. General Information," p. 235, for its availability.

Keep the insulin in a cool place. Although it doesn't have to be refrigerated, it should never be placed where it can overheat or freeze.

Disposable insulin syringes may be used again, despite what you've heard or read—just put the needle cap back on, after the first usage.

In other countries, your child's brand of insulin will probably be available but it may be called something else, so check with the manufacturer of the insulin to see if that's true of your brand. For instance, Novo brand of regular insulin is called Actrapid in various parts of the world. Insulin comes in varying strengths in different parts of the world also. In the United States, it's almost always prescribed in U-100 strength. That, translated, means there are 100 units of insulin per cubic centimeter (cc) of fluid. In some countries, insulin is still prescribed in U-40 and U-80 strengths (40 or 80 units of insulin per cubic centimeter of fluid). You must use a syringe that corresponds with your insulin—a U-100 syringe for U-100 insulin and a U-40 syringe for U-40 insulin. Syringes are usually color coded to match the insulin bottles. Be careful about the unit markings on the syringe you use. The U-100 syringes are available in 50-unit sizes for people who take very small doses. In the 50-unit size, each line on the syringe measures one unit. In the 100-unit size, each line measures two units. Keep this in mind: a unit of insulin remains the same, no matter what strength insulin you're using. A unit of one strength is interchangeable with a unit of any other strength: it is as strong and lowers blood sugar in the same way. What's different is the amount of liquid that holds the insulin. One unit of U-40 has more *volume* than one unit of U-80 or U-100, but the strength of the one unit is exactly the same. You must check with the manufacturer of the insulin to see how to translate one strength to another and still keep the same unit dosage if you are used to taking U-100 strength but can only find U-40 or U-80 strengths in the country you're visiting. If you take along your own insulin, try to take an insulated container for it, to protect against temperature extremes.

Remember to take a note from your doctor (plus extra prescriptions) that describes your child's diabetes and the accoutrements—the needles, syringes, insulin, and other medications you may be carrying. This is essential if you're traveling in another country where local officials and/or Customs agents get *very* nervous whenever they spot "shooting-up" equipment. It doesn't matter if you're a mother with a halo, either. A whole lot of people may not love you if they think you're threatening the morals of their country.

Getting There

If you're traveling by plane, check into special diabetic meals served by airlines and order in advance. On board, tell the stewardess that your child has diabetes, and she'll try to serve at your regular mealtimes.

—Time zone confusion? If you're crossing time zones, keep your watch at your own time zone. Once you've arrived at your destination, if it's not time for an injection and your child wants to sleep—let him. If on awakening, it's been more than twenty-four hours since his last shot, give him a few extra units of insulin (regular). If less than twenty-four hours have passed, give less intermediate-acting insulin, since some of yesterday's dosage is still in the bloodstream. After this injection, set your watch to the time of the place you're in and stay on schedule with your injections.

—It's a good idea to encourage your youngster to walk up and down the aisles every half hour or so, or to straighten her legs and bend and stretch them doing in-seat exercises.

—If your schedule calls for an in-flight injection for your child, the American Diabetes Association suggests you put less air in the insulin bottle (maybe half as much as the number of units you intend to draw out) because there's more pressure in the insulin bottle than in the plane's atmosphere at altitudes over 10,000 feet.

—If your child is inclined toward motion sickness, administer an anti-emetic pill or suppository at least four hours before departure. And take another if nausea occurs in spite of the first pill. Ask your doctor what's the newest and best of these on the market.

And Remember . . .

—You will need an ID. It was not so important when your baby was a baby, but now that he/she is reasonably independent, identification is always necessary. The JDF gives out simple ID cards, but these may be overlooked in the hysteria of an insulin reaction. When traveling—and anytime, actually—the special *Medic-Alert* necklace or bracelet gives up-to-date information that you have provided for your child's computerized medical files, besides informing anyone on the scene that your youngster has diabetes. Applications for these IDs are available from Medic-Alert, Turlock, California 95380 (209-634-4917), or you can write to the American Medical Association, 535 North Dearborn Street, Chicago, Illinois 60610 for a list of other organizations that supply this identification material.

—Get any necessary vaccinations. Do this as least several weeks before you plan to leave so that any reactions will not cause problems during the trip.

—Shoe smarts. New shoes are great, but remember to break them in before the trip. Blisters and foot irritations are a special problem for people with diabetes. Also, take along some foot powder for your child and some nice, cushiony socks.

—Be ready to answer questions at Customs if you travel abroad. Show the identification that says your child has diabetes. Be prepared with a prescription for insulin, extra syringes, and doctors' names in other countries, which you can obtain from the JDF chapter in your community.

While You're There Whooping It Up—And You Overdo

Here's how to say, "I am a diabetic," "Please get me a doctor," and "Sugar or orange juice, please" in four different languages.

I am a diabetic

FRENCH: Je suis diabétique
SPANISH: Yo soy diabético
GERMAN: Ich bin zuckerkrank
ITALIAN: Io sono diabético

Please get me a doctor

FRENCH: Allez chercher un médecin, s'il vous plaît
SPANISH: Haga me el favor de llamar al medico
GERMAN: Rufen Sie bitte einen Arzt
ITALIAN: Per favore chiami un dottor

Sugar or orange juice, please

FRENCH: Sucre ou jus d'orange, s'il vous plaît
SPANISH: Azucar o un vaso de jugo de naranja, por favor
GERMAN: Zucker oder Orangensaft, bitte
ITALIAN: Succhero o succo di arancia, per favore

But unless you're proficient with the language, don't try to be a star and *say* any of this, they'll never understand you. Just whip out the handy card on which you've printed everything, and point to the appropriate phrase.

Some other handy words . . .

Pharmacy (drugstore)	Insulin
FRENCH: pharmacie	FRENCH: insuline
SPANISH: farmacia	SPANISH: insulina
GERMAN: apotheke	GERMAN: insulin
ITALIAN: farmacia	ITALIAN: insulina

Syringe
FRENCH: seringue
SPANISH: jeringa
GERMAN: Spritze
ITALIAN: siringa

Needle
FRENCH: aiguille
SPANISH: aguja
GERMAN: Nadel
ITALIAN: ago

Alcohol
FRENCH: alcool
SPANISH: alcohol
GERMAN: Alkohol
ITALIAN: alcool

Cotton
FRENCH: coton
SPANISH: algodón
GERMAN: Baumwölle
ITALIAN: cotone

Food
FRENCH: nourriture
SPANISH: alimento
GERMAN: Nahrung
ITALIAN: cibo

TIP: In Great Britain, a pharmacist is known as a chemist and cotton is called cotton wool.

Eating and Drinking

Eating unfamiliar or tainted foods or drinking local water that may not have been purified or even boiled may create digestion problems. Certain foods in certain countries, notably South or Central America, Asia, or Africa, are very often responsible. *Avoid* the local water (bottled drinking water is available almost everywhere), raw meats, milk products, ice cubes, lettuce or other leafy vegetables.

Some Further Pointers

—Adjust your child's food and insulin intake accordingly if you play much harder on vacation. Never allow him/her to swim, ski, hike, or bike alone in case of an insulin reaction. Lee's son Larry had an insulin reaction while he was surfing and certainly would have been lost if a "buddy" was not nearby.

—Before any special exertion like water skiing or swimming, have your child eat some fruit or crackers or ice cream (if you're sure that the ice cream is good) to avoid a reaction.

—Late nights are okay, and so is oversleeping, actually. If you end up sleeping late and missing breakfast, give less insulin in that first shot. If you travel to a country where dinner is fashionably late, you can either give a smaller dose of insulin in the morning and an extra small dose before bedtime; or you can give the usual morning shot and the major part of the carbohydrates normally taken at six o'clock, and the rest of the dinner (minus the carbohydrates) at the later hour.

—It's your responsibility to figure out the caloric and carbohydrate exchange in terms of the new foods in the new places. The body's cells craving the proper amount of energy don't know when it's Tuesday and you're in Hawaii eating mangos (which are loaded with sugar). So get into the habit of checking blood sugar or urine quite often to see if it is positive for sugar.

—You're not even sure that the bottled water is so pure? Brush teeth with Coca-Cola.

—Wash glasses with *hot*, not cold water. Bring along straws to drink directly from commercial soda bottles. If you must have cold liquids, put ice around a bottle rather than in it.

—Watch out for sunburn, fluid loss (from more sun and more activity), and poison-ivy type agonies. One mother we know was sure her son was having an insulin reaction because he was weak and sweaty; all he was having was far too much sun and games.

—Most of all, relax, have a ball, and start planning the next trip on the way home.

NOTE: Most countries around the world have organizations comparable to the Juvenile Diabetes Foundation. If you write to the International Diabetes Federation, 3–6 Alfred Place, London WCIE 7EE, England, you can get the names of diabetes specialists all over the world. JDF can get you such names, also. Be prepared with the names of physicians before you leave, so you'll be all ready if an emergency crops up. You may be interested in visiting some of the newest research facilities to see, first hand, what the latest developments in diabetes research are. JDF can tell you where such centers exist. In a serious emergency, if you've lost all your carefully obtained names, call the United States Embassy in a foreign country for help. Of course, if your travel has taken you to Squeedonk, U.S.A., calling the embassy is stretching it a bit. Just call the Squeedonk Diabetes Association for a doctor experienced in diabetes care. And don't panic. If you yourself are knowledgeable about your child's disease, you can probably handle most situations. And if you can't, all major hotels have access to medical assistance.

TIP: Don't overreact to a few higher than normal sugar readings, but watch for trends of high or low readings and ketones in the urine.

Okay, Let's do it again ... Have you got
- syringes?
- swabs?
- more than enough insulin, at least a week's worth more?
- urine-testing and/or blood-testing supplies for glucose and ketones?
- a note from your doctor; a prescription for insulin and other medications?
- an ID tag that includes child's regular dosage of insulin, the times, and type you use?
- carbohydrate snacks?
- glucagon, Instant Glucose, cake gels, honey, or Monogel?
- motion sickness medication and anti-diarrhetic medication?

FAST FOOD

McDiabetes—Have It Your Way

This is the age when the fast food frenzies start. Can your child stop into McDonald's or Burger King, with the rest of the gang? Sure! But he's got to do it with thought.

Instead of a Big Mac, a hamburger, cheeseburger, or fish filet sandwich is his best bet. A shake is ignored in favor of a diet soda or low-fat milk. If he has half a hamburger, he can have some french fries. Whatever he chooses, he has to be aware of empty calories and concentrated carbohydrates and sugars. Most fast food places have salad bars now.

If it's a place for a chicken dinner that the gang chooses, have your child remove the batter-coated skin of the chicken and ignore the mayonnaise-loaded coleslaw. Cut back on what's given: for instance, if two or three pieces of fish come with the fish and chips, only have one or two pieces, removing the covering.

Pizza? It's not bad at all, often providing a well-balanced meal that includes vegetables, meat, dairy, and bread products all in one. Just go easy is the message.

Look for the food that's not fried or drowned in sauce, oil, or mayonnaise. Look for fast foods that don't have double bread allotments like Big Macs or Super Subs. Look for fresh fruit juices—not fruit "drinks," which have sugar added.

And think about *when* your child is visiting these fast food places. A hamburger with half a roll and a diet soda might be okay during a time when he usually has a snack; an order of a Big Mac or a Whopper and french fries between regular meals might be *terrible* for diabetes management.

Any youngster must feel "part of the crowd" when the crowd opts for eating out. That's as essential for his emotional growth as controlling blood sugar is for his physical well-being. So—don't be the kind of parent who says No automatically out of fear and lack of education. Adjustments can be made in almost every area, including food; properly briefed, your child can go along with his peers, if he uses his head.

Because fast food stopovers are probably inevitable, your child ought to learn about the probable calorie exchanges he'll have to calculate mentally. Usually, the chains show remarkable uniformity in their portion sizes and their nutritional offerings, so it's really not too difficult to make fast food exchanges once in a while. We include below a chart that lists the approximate values of most of the foods, or types of foods, found in the fast food restaurants to help you make some intelligent exchange choices. It's not necessary for your child to carry the chart around in preparation for a fast trip to Burger King; on the other hand, it's a wise move to go over it with him/her in advance of such trips, so that some speedy calculations in the head can be made when the moment comes.

This is a good time to discuss eating in general. Although opinion varies as to whether children with diabetes ought to be on absolutely prescribed diets as opposed to an "unmeasured" diet, common sense and many doctors are beginning to support the unmeasured diet. Dr. Robert Kaye is the chief of Pediatric Medicine at Hahnemann Hospital in Philadelphia, and he feels strongly about this diet business. "What the average child requires is always within a range," he maintains, "and diet should always be placed at a level that is comfortable for the kid. If a young person is not obese and is well nourished at a proper weight, he no doubt has an inner mechanism that tells him how to control his weight—and that should be respected. Although a nutritionally sound diet makes a lot of sense, it is physiologically sound to permit some flexibility in the daily caloric intake."

Children in control of their blood sugar should be permitted to decide the amount of food they eat, which can vary as they grow or even from day to day. Nutritionists can help give guidelines about exchange possibilities, but every child ought to be encouraged to be responsible, as soon as possible, for his/her own eating choices. And that may or may not include an occasional "junk food" binge.

Sugarless Foods—A Blessing? Well, Maybe

If you're not careful, sugarless foods may well be a punch in the diabetes control instead of a blessing. In a world where your child is denied the ordinary snacks, it does seem a blessing to have diet foods to offer as an alternative. Yet the diet or "artificial sweetener foods" may not be acceptable for the child with diabetes at all. Many of the terms on the label that

NUTRITIONAL VALUES OF FAST FOODS AND THEIR EXCHANGE VALUES*

	\	NUTRITIONAL VALUES			EXCHANGES		
	CAL.	CARB. (grams)	PRO (grams)	FAT (grams)	BREAD	MEAT (medium)	FAT
LONG JOHN SILVER							
Fish, chips, coleslaw							
3-piece dinner	1190	100	55	63	7	6	7
2-piece dinner	955	89	38	50	6	3½	6
McDONALD'S							
Hamburger	260	31	14	9	1½	1	1½
Cheeseburger	306	31	16	13	2	2	1
Quarter Pounder	418	33	26	21	2	3	1
Quarter Pounder with cheese	518	34	31	29	2½	3½	2
Big Mac	550	44	21	32	3	2	4
Filet-O-Fish	402	34	15	23	2½	1½	3
French fries	211	26	3	11	2	—	2
Egg McMuffin	352	26	18	20	2	2	2
Pork sausage	184	trace	9	17	—	1	2½
Scrambled eggs	162	2	12	12	—	1½	1
Shake, chocolate	364	60	11	9	4	½	1
PIZZA HUT							
Cheese pizza							
individual							
thick crust	1030	143	71	19	9½	6	—
thin crust	1005	128	61	28	8½	6	—
½ of 13-inch							
thick crust	900	113	65	21	7½	6	—
thin crust	850	103	50	26	7	5	—
1 slice (⅛ of pie)	225	26	12½	6½	2	2	—
½ of 15-inch							
thick crust	1200	148	83	31	10	7	—
thin crust	1150	144	66	35	9½	7	—
SUBMARINE HERO GRINDER							
8-inch sandwich							
Italian cold cuts	620	60	36	26	4	4	1
Roast beef	600	55	46	22	3½	5	—
Tuna	700	55	41	34	3½	5	2
TACO BELL							
Bean Burrito	343	48	11	12	3	1	2
Beef Burrito	466	37	30	21	2½	3½	½
Beefy Tostada	291	21	19	15	1½	2½	½
Bellbeefer	221	23	15	7	1½	2	—
Bellbeefer with cheese	278	23	19	12	1½	2	½
Burrito Supreme	457	43	21	22	3	2	2½
Combination Burrito	404	43	21	16	3	2	1
Enchirito	454	42	25	21	3	3	1½
Pintos 'n Cheese	168	21	11	5	1½	1	—
Taco	186	14	15	8	1	2	—
Tostada	179	25	9	6	2	1	—

*Reprinted with permission from *Diabetes Forecast*, Copyright © 1979 by the American Diabetes Association.

seem to make the food safe from sugar may be just another word for sugar itself. For instance, *sucrose* is sugar. *Fructose* is, true, a type of sugar that does not require insulin for its metabolism, but, says Dr. Fredda Ginsberg-Fellner, because it still converts to glucose in the body, it's exactly like eating any other kind of sugar. Somewhat safer are sugar substitutes like *sorbitol, mannitol,* or *xylitol,* which are sugar alcohols that are converted to glucose but absorbed into the bloodstream much more slowly. Handled in small amounts, they're less likely to cause a serious blood sugar rise. Still, says Dr. Ginsberg-Fellner, "we don't know the long-range results of this diet stuff, so it must be used in moderation. No more than two diet sodas a day, for instance, and less if you have anything else with sorbitol, mannitol, xylitol, or even saccharine in it. As a matter of fact, these substances may give stomach cramps or diarrhea to many."

Furthermore, it's essential to keep in mind that some sweeteners are caloric as opposed to non-caloric saccharine. Sweeteners that sound healthy but are highly caloric and filled with glucose are honey, carob powder, maltose, and corn or maple syrups.

Saccharine is truly a non-caloric sweetener that contains no carbohydrates. It's genuinely sugar-free.

So, remember to read labels. Anything that has an ingredient that ends in *-ose,* such as *lactose* or *dextrose,* is almost surely a sugar product. Here's an interesting tip. If the sweetener's position(s) in the list of ingredients is on top of the list, it's the ingredient used in the largest amount by weight. Check with your physician to see if it's non-caloric, non-sugar, and safe. If a manufacturer says the product is sugar-free, he usually means no *sucrose* has been added; but other sugars may well have been added.

And go easy on the sorbitol, mannitol, and xylitol products.

OTHER IMPORTANT THINGS TO CONSIDER

Barefoot Blues

There's something about young people and walking around barefoot that seem to go together. Although Dr. Ginsberg-Fellner says cuts and bruises heal on a diabetic youngster with good blood sugar control about the same as they heal in any other youngster, both the bottoms of the feet and the knees are, once cut or bruised, hard places to heal. Also, they're very prone to develop infections. So try to convince that barefoot kid of yours to wear some kind of foot covering, and if she does cut herself in any of these places, to keep it scrupulously clean. Naturally, it goes without saying that if your youngster's blood sugar is not in good control, you must watch for infection particularly carefully.

Dear Sibling—or I'm Not My Brother's Keeper

Well, yes you are, in a way. If your brother has diabetes and he has an insulin reaction, you sure ought to know what to do about it. In that way, you are his keeper even though his diabetes is not your responsibility. And even though you're mightily tempted, you do have to learn that it's pretty crummy to taunt your brother with the anchovy pizza or the hot fudge sundae when you're pigging out. And though it's hard, you have to remember that if you feel unspeakable rage at your parents, who seem to give him all the attention, he didn't ask to have that miserable disease and it's really not his fault that they seem to be ignoring your needs. The best thing you can do about *that* is to talk with them, one quiet evening, and explain how you need more than you're getting from them.

And did you ever feel guilty that it's your brother who got the disease and not you? Well, don't. Heredity is capricious and you'll have to pay your dues in something else, don't worry: for instance, did you ever notice how much nicer his nose is than yours? Sure you have. Now you don't have to feel guilty any more, right? You're getting your inherited angst in the Big Nose Department. Or the Fatness Department. Which, let's face it, isn't as bad as diabetes, but it counts for something.

Look, you hate this intruder of a disease in your family, and it does make a lot of changes in the way you eat and live, but face it—the more casually you accept the differences, the more the same as you your brother will be. Naturally, your parents ought to set the tone of the family. You need glasses, he needs insulin, she needs tutoring for math. Differences in a family abound, and we're betting on you: you can handle them! BE your brother's keeper out of love, and he'll be yours for the same reason.

Be Your Own Boss

If you'll hear it once, you'll hear it a thousand times over the years: "It's his diabetes, not yours." And it's true. Although parents should be around for counseling and emotional succor into a child's young adulthood, certainly, the sooner your youngster begins to claim the responsibilities and chores of diabetes management, the better it is for all of you. And you can't give the whole shebang to your kid on a silver platter one day when he looks particularly mature. Transferring management has to be a gradual procedure, starting when very young.

In the early years, if your child was diagnosed before four, accepting management may mean swabbing an injection site with alcohol or dipping a Diastix into urine to test for sugar or deciding which site is to be used for injection. As capability grows, responsibilities must increase. We know five-year-olds who give themselves injections and measure (with supervision) proper doses of insulin all by themselves. Certainly, as soon as a child starts school, he/she has to understand about what's a no-no in terms of food and overexertion. If Jason's classmate wants to trade his own sugar-bombed Yankee Doodle snack for Jason's nice healthy apple, a little voice in Jason's head has to go off saying, "No way, buddy!" A thousand little voices saying No in *your* head don't do Jason one bit of good when he's not tied to your apron strings.

The very best way to maintain equilibrium in your family and in all your psyches is to allow your child with diabetes as much self-supervision as possible. Unless he learns to deal with his own disease, he can never have a sleep-over date, never go away with the team for a game, never go to camp, never really go to school successfully. What's more, it gets worse. Jason's wife is not going to be thrilled when you move in to supervise his lunches.

So start young. With pride and self-assurance, your little one will be able to take care of himself—with you around, naturally, to help with the big decisions. When you hand over diabetes control, you hand over his emotional and physical well-being.

$$$ and Cents

This whole thing costs money—a lot. But there are ways to offset expenses, and the best is to check with other parents and with your local JDF for suggestions. To start you off, remember that most dealers, including drugstores, etc., are willing to negotiate prices if you're really a steady customer. Sometimes you can get up to a 15 percent discount from list prices. Major medical insurance covers much of the cost of the paraphernalia used in diabetes management (if prescribed by a physician) like blood- and urine-testing equipment. Look into the SSI (Supplemental Security Income) program, which gives federal funds in the form of monthly cash payments to disabled people who have very limited funds and assets. To get information, request HEW Publication No. (SSA) 78-11039 (SSI for Disabled or Blind Children) from a Social Security office. Look into accident, health, hospitalization *group* insurance plans that can be obtained at no extra premium. And remember to claim medical expenses, trips to the doctor if they require traveling expenses, and other deductible items on your income tax returns. Check with an accountant or your local JDF chapter to get a list of exactly what's deductible.

Depression

Can a ten-year-old be profoundly depressed? It's no good ignoring the problem, because the answer is Yes. Although many children become depressed over many things, it's not so crazy to think that a child with diabetes has good reason to be sad or upset. First of all, he's got to remember to DO so many things. Then, he's got to think about the future, his mortality, if you will, a subject that rarely crosses the mind of most ten-year-olds, who think they're invincible. It's very hard for a ten-year-old really to get it into his head that if he doesn't exercise control now—in his ten-year-old-ness—when he's forty, he may be having visual problems. That's pretty far in the future, and no wonder if it's a downer when the realization finally hits home. Dr. M. Kovacs, an associate professor of psychiatry at the University of Pittsburgh Medical School, is conducting a long-term study of depression in children. If the child feels that having diabetes is a terrible disruption, Dr. Kovacs discovered, he or she is more likely to become quite saddened than the child who looks upon the disease as a manageable annoyance. One solution to the problem that seems to have been effective is for a depressed child is "go out and become very good at something."

It makes sense. Sure, you can drag the kid off to therapy for a whole lot of dollars a session, and that's often a super way for anyone to get in touch with her inner turmoil; but it's perhaps even more satisfying to become an expert at something. Everybody loves an expert and admires him/her. It raises the self-esteem 10 million percent. It gives you a skill for the rest of your life. It may even make you big bucks in the future. But for now, right now, learning to be as good as could be in one thing, ANYthing, is a road to popularity, self-assurance, and a fine route out of depression.

What could the thing be? Well, sports for starters. Your child could be a star tennis player, basketball person, swimmer, with the proper lessons and practice. Talk to the coach at school, to the pro in your neighborhood, and encourage an athletically minded child to be wonderful at something. Naturally, this does *not* mean being one of those parents who is visibly crestfallen when the point for the team is lost. Developing the expertise is your child's ego, not yours. Perhaps there's a hint of some skill in art or music or creative writing. Student magazines can be started with some adult direction, artistic talent can be encouraged, small businesses can be begun (you better believe it) before a child even enters high school.

The point is to help your child think of something that, with practice and concentration, he can become super at. You may be helping him find a direction for the rest of his life, or you may be just helping to develop a skill that will ease him over the bad times of this disease—and with adolescence on the horizon, the bad times are not far away: the times when worries about womanliness/manliness are strongest, the time of natural rebellions. Dr. Kovacs might have just hit upon the one thing that makes a difference when a child is feeling down, and that is feeling superior at some skill. It helps. It's worth a shot. Even if a star is not exactly born, trying to become an expert at something tends to push diabetes into the background of life. At the same time, it propels the *whole* child into the foreground.

THE UNSPEAKABLE THOUGHTS

During the course of writing this book, we've sat around for uncountable hours with kids of every age—just rapping and finding out what bugs them most about having diabetes. It might be a good idea for you to consider some of their responses because often you're not hearing what your kid is feeling but can't or won't say out loud. If you feel that any of these musings are relevant to your child, perhaps you might open up the subject somehow and make it easier for the fears to be expressed, and thus banished. The following exchanges took place during a rap session in which Kevin (age eleven), Sarah (age ten), Eliezer (age nine), Sue (age eleven), and Barney (age seven) took part.

Lee: "Okay, how did you feel when you first found out you had diabetes?"

"I felt scared," says Eliezer. "I didn't know what was coming next. They were all running around in the hospital doing things and nobody told me what was happening."

"I thought really that maybe I would die," says Sue. "My mother was crying and she *never* cries."

Lee: "And now, how do you feel about the disease? Do you ever feel angry? Or maybe that you made it happen to yourself because you did something wrong?"

"Yes, yes—that's right!" says Kevin. "I've always thought, I still think I do, that maybe if I didn't eat so much candy like my mother always told me, that this wouldn't have happened. You know she never knew *how* much candy I really ate. I used to buy some after school every day . . ."

Lee: "You know, you can't get diabetes because you were bad or because you ate too much sugar or because of anything wrong you did. It just doesn't work that way. Still, Kevin, a lot of kids feel the way you do . . ."

Barney, the littlest, chimes in with: "I can't have candy at a birthday party, I can't sleep at my friend's, I can't not have shots, I hate diabetes . . ."

Sarah reaches out to hug Barney. "Me, too, Barney," she says. "I hate it like poison, too."

"Sometimes I feel that I want to hit my Dad, when he comes near me with those needles," says Sue. "I know he has to do it but I still get mad at him. I should learn to do it myself, he says, and I'm scared to."

Lee: "Do you ever have any embarrassing moments? Is there something about diabetes that's worse than any other thing?"

Sarah, for the first time, speaks in a whisper. "Yes," she says. The whole group leans forward to hear. "I hate it when my mother says that I shouldn't tell anybody about it—my friends, I mean. I always feel as if I've got this awful *secret* and I'd die if anyone found out. My mother says that parents might not let their kids play with me if everyone knew. And the other day, I felt a little shocky while we were having this fair in our back-yard; I got so dizzy, and I wanted to tell my friend to get me some candy, but then, she would have been suspicious. Lucky, my mother came out just then with some orange juice. I felt embarrassed."

Lee: "Do any of the rest of you feel you shouldn't tell anyone? Wouldn't you feel *easier* sharing this? It's not anything to be ashamed of, you know. What if you had a broken finger, would you mention it?"

"It's not me that doesn't want to tell," whispers Sarah. "It's my mother."

Sue says, "I tell everybody. Why shouldn't I? My friends all know and everybody plays with me just the same."

Eliezer says, "You know what embarrasses me? One of my friends called me a junky freak. He says that only junky freaks shoot up like I do."

Sue can't stand it, and comes in with "Your friend is a weirdo freak, you know that? And he's also a stupid."

Conversations and reachings out, like this, seem to be a priceless balm to the unvoiced guilt feelings and fears of everybody—and that includes adults. An hour of this kind of thing often saves twenty hours in the psychiatrist's office. Somehow, group dynamics sweep a lot of cobwebs out of the closet where too many people stash their diabetes. JDF people can arrange such group sessions for parents or for children, to be held separately or together. Give it a try!

THE "DO YOU WANT TO KNOW WHAT WE DO?" SECTION

There is nothing, literally nothing, that helps more than hearing how the other guys do it. Here are some real suggestions from real people that have helped to get the child with diabetes safely and happily (not to mention inexpensively) through the day. If you can find one suggestion that saves money or makes your life immeasurably easier, it's worth the price of this book. Right? Right!

—Cut Chemstrips into thirds. They're expensive and there's no need to use the whole strip.

—Prick the fingers (when testing) on the inside edges near the nail, not on the plush pad which you need to push, to write, to play piano, or pick up objects. It hurts less on that inside edge because the nerves seem far less sensitive there.

—Insulin feels better if it's allowed to warm to room temperature in the syringe before injecting.

—I always keep a snack in the glove compartment of my car in case of a flat tire, traffic jam, or who knows what! Flip-top orange or apple juice cans take up little room and are always available in time of need. The other day, my son's friend looked a little funny to me although everyone else seemed to notice nothing. I raced to my glove compartment, got him a can of orange juice, and sure enough, headed off a serious insulin reaction in a kid who has never told anyone about his diabetes. Living with the disease sure makes you observant of other people's symptoms! After heavy game playing on the way home, my son is grateful for the cans just to "get himself together . . ."

—I always hang the disposable syringe in a medicine bottle filled with alcohol in the bathroom. It can be reused until it's no longer sharp, and the technique is medically sound if it's being used only by one person.

—We keep an exerciser machine in the bedroom for my son. In the winter when there's a drop in physical activity, it's terrific to keep that blood sugar down. Often, also, after a heavy dinner or a high sugar reading, he'll ride for twenty minutes while watching TV. It works!

—I spend time at the beginning of each school year with the other mothers in my daughter's car pool. I explain diabetes to them and give them (a) printed information with "signs to watch for reactions"; and (b) a dozen sugar cubes in a plastic bag to be kept in each mother's glove compartment. I explain that in the event of a flat tire, traffic jam, snow emergency, etc., they will be prepared for any reaction from my daughter. This is especially important at twelve noon when nursery school lets out and an important meal is coming up. Now that my daughter carries a school bag, I include the same emergency packet with emergency information about whom to contact, what to do, and—of course—her name and address.

—I found that my baby daughter loved eating out in a restaurant. She was always a crummy eater, and since I was desperate to get lunch into her (her insulin would peak in the afternoon), it was McDonald's for us for a burger and fries. It cost a little more but it was worth the compromise in my frustration-alleviation, alone.

—For a snack that's easily carried around by a child, try dried apple chunks

(Weight-Watchers is one brand equal to one fruit exchange).

—Watch out for very hot, humid days. Reactions for my child always seem more likely on these days.

—We allow Sharon to "trick or treat" on Halloween and then offer to trade with her for the candy she cannot eat. Boxes of raisins, peanuts, sugarless gum are good trades that she particularly loves!

—Maple syrup is a terrific fast sugar source; when it comes in the spout bottle, it's easy to use in an emergency.

—You can test the amount of sugar in prepared baby foods with a Tes-Tape dunked into the food.

—My nursery schooler knows there's always a food or sugar snack waiting for her in the nurse's office if she feels "shocky."

—I would always panic when my child was ill because I knew I had to get enough sugar down him to recover the insulin shock—or to quickly bring him out of an insulin reaction. Then I discovered those baby-ice-cube trays (¼ inch by ¼ inch size). I'd freeze Coke or ginger ale in them and my child was always willing to chew them even when he didn't feel like eating anything else. It also does away with forcing down the MonoGel or Cake Mate stuff my child always objected to. You can freeze Coke ice-pops in the plastic pop containers and have them on hand for the older child.

—Each teacher has in her desk a package of Kraft Cheese and Crackers or Peanut Butter Crackers (one meat and one bread exchange). They come sealed and stay fresh, and the teachers know to give him the orange juice if he feels shocky, followed by a protein and a carbohydrate. He also uses them for extra pick-ups if he's going to have a strenuous gym class or he's playing a softball game that runs into extra time, causing him to delay or miss lunch.

—Things that are great to carry on trips or inconvenient places are Planters nuts in small packages (fat exchanges) and variety packs of chips, Doritos, pretzels, Cheetos, etc., which are used as bread exchanges.

—Sweet 'n Low puts out packages of individual servings of iced tea mix as well as flavored drink packets. When you can't get a diet soda, you can always get a glass of water and ice to make this free exchange.

—You don't have to be on a serious trip to carry prescriptions in your glove compartment for needles and insulin, and the doctor's phone number.

You never know when you'll need to purchase them anytime you're out on the road.

—After my daughter was diagnosed, and when we came home from the hospital, we made up a chart which we still use variations of ten years later. It's a rotation chart and it shows the front and back of her legs and arms, and her buttocks. There are about six sites on the front and back of each leg, arm, and buttock, and we note every injection in every site. At the moment, we're going about twenty-four to twenty-eight days before we come back to the same site, and it sure prevents the denting of the skin that occurs from overusing the same sites.

—I always keep a flip-top can of juice on top of my baby's dresser, along with the baby powder and creams. When minutes count (especially in the middle of the night), it's helpful not to have to run to the kitchen for a quick sugar fix. I also carry a ¼ ounce box of raisins (exactly one fruit exchange) and prewrapped packages of saltines in my handbag for a quick snack in an unexpected delay. Cake gel in a squeeze tube is always to be found in my purse in case my child is past the point of being able to drink or eat.

—As soon as my child was able to read, I involved her in label reading at the grocery store and in cooking. Cooking together can be a positive approach to proper food preparation and consumption, as well as companionship.

—A terrific tout for me has been keeping the syringes, etc., in a pretty box: It gives a more cheerful, non-clinical aura to injections.

—I use the fact that we have to wake up earlier than anyone else on weekends for injections to provide a good, cozy time for family breakfasts together. Our family is the only one on the block that breakfasts together on Saturdays and Sundays, and we usually end up with friends whose own parents are sleeping through a marvelous time for togetherness.

—The Cake Mate icing is neat and portable for coaches' pockets, teachers' desks, and night stand drawers. I distribute several tubes at the beginning of each school year to everyone who will come actively into my child's life.

—Individual alcohol swabs get expensive! I use a bottle of alcohol and tissues or toilet paper to cleanse injection areas. It lasts longer and is much more economical.

—This tip may not work for all age groups, or even all children, but I'm sure it has contributed to my own son's adjustment to having diabetes. The first day back at school after being diagnosed, and again at the beginning of the new school year, my son gave a short report to his class about diabetes. He brought in a piece of plywood on which he had attached a syringe, some insulin in a bottle, blood- and urine-testing equipment, and a copy of his diet plan. He told the kids what diabetes is, described insulin reactions, explained that diabetes is not contagious, and outlined his diet.

When Jeff first told me that he wanted to do this, I wasn't sure it was a good idea. I thought it might single him out as being "different" and the children might tease him. Instead, the report had the opposite effect. Now that the children understand what diabetes is and see that Jeff is comfortable with it, they also are comfortable. On birthdays when parents send in cupcakes or other sweets, they always seem to include some sugarless gum or baseball cards for Jeff. *I* have an added sense of security knowing that his friends know the symptoms of a reaction and that he always has Lifesavers in his pocket. They don't even seem to mind that he's allowed to eat snacks during the school day; in fact, they've reminded him twice to remember to take his snack off the bus during field trips. This cuts out an awful lot of subterfuge and guilt that other kids seem to experience as they "leave the room" for their snacks. Jeff's openness about diabetes has helped everyone with whom he comes in contact to feel relaxed and totally normal about him.

3 SUGAR TEENS

THE WORST OF TIMES

"It was the best of times, it was the worst of times," wrote Dickens. Ask the doctor or the parents of an adolescent with diabetes and they'll change the refrain to,"It was the worst of times, it was the worst of times, it was the very worst of times."

Everything seems to conspire against proper control for the teenager and there are moments when even once-loving adolescents and adults would seriously consider strangling each other. Combine a serious disease that requires constant self-monitoring with the physical tumults and emotional insurrections of adolescence and you usually get mayhem.

But the doctor told you there's no reason why it shouldn't be a "normal" adolescence? You and the doctor can tell that teenager till you're all blue in the face that she's having a "normal" adolescence and it won't work. If you keep insisting upon your point, at best, you're being patronizing, and at worst, a true pain and not to be trusted. It's not normal to have to worry about complications that may occur when you're fifty, at sixteen. It's not normal to be thinking about your very mortality when adolescents, by nature, tend to suspect they'll go on forever. It's not normal to be hassling with blood samples and urine tests, it's not normal to say No to a hot fudge sundae, and it's sure as heck not normal never to be able to sleep late when you're sixteen. So don't talk "normal" to the adolescent with diabetes if you want her to hear you. Talk honesty.

Honesty says that the youngster with diabetes will have many more difficult and frustrating times than the youngster without the disease; but honesty also says that she can lead as full, sweet, and productive a life as any other kid. That is the truth. That is NOT being patronizing. You and the adolescent in your life have surely read the statistics about shorter life spans and complicating disabilities and, make no mistake, they will be very real for some. They are not crazy numbers made up by sadistic minds. But the good news is that you happen to be living at a crucial turning point and the statistics have not yet caught up with the reality. Methods of testing and caring for diabetes have so improved during the last couple of years that the statistics may be rewritten soon.

The fact is that many people do beat the odds. If you control your disease and don't let it control you, there's a whole new ballgame out there. The experts, the *real* experts, are much encouraged by what's happening. Dr. Fredda Ginsberg-Fellner, who as we said earlier is director of the Division of Pediatric Endocrinolgy and Metabolism at the Mount Sinai School of Medicine in New York, stated that it is absolutely reasonable to assume you can have a long life, relatively free of complications, if you're quite careful with your diabetes control. Dr. Leo Krall, chief of Education at the well-known Joslin Diabetes Foundation in Boston, Massachusetts, says that "now, there's real good news—such exciting hope. A short time ago we'd have given an insulin-dependent diabetic who lived for twenty-five years after diagnosis a parade. Now we have people coming into Joslin who have survived fifty and many more years and no one pays too much attention to them. More important, actually, is that we're on the *verge* of even greater discoveries than those in the last five or ten years that have made all this possible."

So you can almost write the script yourself. If you happen to be a teenager with diabetes, if you go to hell with yourself over the next few years, you can't make it magically better after you hit twenty-one. Being sloppy with control, right now, this very minute, will compromise your physical state for the rest of your life. You are still growing, your body is producing massive hormonal changes, and what you do now really sets the stage for the life performance. A "screw it, I'll worry about the whole thing when I'm thirty-two" attitude may preclude your ever reaching thirty-two. On the other hand, if you exercise *reasonable* care and good judgment (no one says you have to be perfect), then, even though the taking care is a pain in the butt, it may be making you a promise of a good life.

Dr. Krall puts it this way: "Having diabetes is a little like being on a ship. If you take common sense precautions, you stay high and dry. But if you look down, you can see the ocean forever trying to get into that ship. You can never, ever forget it's there, not when you're eating, traveling, having fun."

Now that's not a normal life, as we said before. But there are worse things. Diabetes doesn't show, for instance. You're not covered with ghastly red spots, you don't wheeze horribly, so the only people who have to know about your disease are those whom you tell. And you have a chance to help yourself—which is more than can be said about many other diseases. Think of it this way: "If one out of two diabetics will develop some of the more serious complications in a lifetime, I'll be the one who doesn't!" Diabetes, under control, doesn't stop you for one minute from working, marrying, having children, having a whole lot of fun.

There's one other thing. Crazy as it sounds, there's something to be said for having the disease. We've seen it happen time and time again and we don't really know why it happens, but it does. It more often than not emerges that young people who have hassled through diabetes turn out to have very special lives. They end up being the presidents of their classes or companies. They end up being somebodies. No kidding. Like Billy Talbert—Davis Cup tennis champion; Mary Tyler Moore—actress; Thomas Edison—inventor; Paul Cézanne—artist; H. G. Wells—writer; George Lucas—*Star Wars* filmmaker; Puccini—composer; Gayle W. McGee—senator. Perhaps it's the effort and the discipline they've needed to develop; perhaps it's the will to do more than just survive, to live and use every moment, that makes them special. We don't really know. All that's clear is that young people with diabetes, instead of being consumed with worry over zits and the latest disco spots, tend to be more original, more mature, more *doing*. Hard knocks don't flatten them. They learn to deal with adversity; they learn to canter instead of plod. They're not lost in the crowd. It's a fine thing to see.

But you know what? If there's a kind of credit, a special bonus that goes along with having the disease, they deserve it. Because it ain't easy.

A Message to Parents

(If you're the kid with the diabetes, don't read this. It will give you too much ammunition to hold over their heads.)

"Let It Be, Let It Be . . ." says the pop song, and if you're the parent of an adolescent with diabetes, you ought to take the lyrics to heart. Rebellion is almost a natural and expected part of growing up because so many teenagers feel the need to assert their adulthood, their growing independence. The trick is to hope the rebellion doesn't compromise the diabetes. Dr. Fredda Ginsberg-Fellner says that when the teenager in your life decides he's *had* it with testing, decides he's *had* it with eating properly or taking his insulin on time, your thinking should go along these lines: I'm not sure I can do anything about it by creating a confrontation, it will be a passing thing if I don't make too much out of it and just let it be, let it be. . .

This doesn't mean that you lean back and watch the teenager irrevocably harm himself. It *does* mean that you nag as little as possible, that you don't expect perfection in every thing, and that you settle for long, horribly dirty hair or sloppy rooms as a personal rebellion as long as your son takes care of his diabetes. It means you say to your kid: "Look, we know you're going to experiment with liquor no matter how we forbid you to do so, so for Pete's sake, if you must drink a little, take a little wine instead of a sugared mixed drink, and for God's sakes, *eat* while you're rebelling with that alcohol."

Let it go, let it go means that *even if you're terrified* that, because no one knows about your son's diabetes at the school dance, he'll have an insulin reaction and die, still you should NOT tell his date or best friend if he doesn't wish to. You will be guilty of the worst kind of betrayal if you do so, and you'll cause a relationship between kid and parents that is hostile and secretive. Let it be, let it be...

The very worst antidotes to an adolescent's carelessness about his self-care are threats, hysteria, or punishments. If you feed the "melodrama of adolescence," as Dr. Charles Weller, director of the Diabetes Research Unit at Grasslands Hospital in New York, says, it leads to "self-pity, which induces the diabetic to try to punish his parents or his girlfriend or his teachers by letting the disease get out of control." A vicious cycle.

A teenager who is expected to measure everything she eats and completely eschew McDonald's when the rest of the crowd lands there may suddenly develop a remarkable preoccupation with some pretty exotic eating habits that are ghastly for diabetes! Stigmata that set teenagers apart from their peers are the end of the world, and if you place unreasonable demands on your adolescent, expect to get back a whole lot of trouble.

If you tell your seventeen-year-old son that it's okay to play football and then deluge him with your own fears, restrictions, and stomach-grippers, you'll not only kill his game but you'll murder his self-confidence and maybe even cause an accident. Let it go, let it go—your own worries, realistic or not, that is.

You don't have to win the argument. You don't have to make the point. Relax. Talk as much as possible, when your child feels like talking, but don't push togetherness if she doesn't. The best thing you can do for your child is to encourage group sessions with other adolescents who have diabetes. Somehow that works to promote common sense better than any parent-pontificating.

And the next time you absolutely feel you have to make a stand and prove a point, ask yourself if it wouldn't be better to let it be, let it be ...

"I'm Mad and I'm Not Going to Take It Any More!"

That's what the star of the movie *Network* yelled out the window at the world to tell of his anger. If you are an adolescent with diabetes, you probably feel like doing the same thing, more often than not.

Having diabetes means having a whole lot of anger. It's not surprising why. First of all, why you? You're such a nice person, a good person, and damn it, you didn't deserve to be chosen for this miserable thing. Then, there are your parents: you can't help it, but they get you angry, too. Either they're just too saintly putting up with the whole thing or you feel their own "why me?" syndrome peeking out even though they try hard not to show it. Then, there's the rest of the world. Some of your friends who know try to understand, but they really don't. They can't understand the *foreverness* of the disease, the fact that you can never let it go or even take a vacation from it. So it gets you angry when they say they completely understand—when they can't.

Doctors and books trying to get you to ventilate your anger (like even this book you're reading right now) irritate you, also. It seems as if they're playing a psychological game with your fragile emotions. It makes you feel so . . . vulnerable. So raw. What's more, crazy as it sounds, seeing their side of it gets you even madder. So what that your parents didn't order a set of needles and a syringe of insulin along with their adolescent, and they may be suffering also. Big deal. And so what that your siblings and friends are veritable pillars of patience and so understanding of your problem: it's not they who get the insulin reactions with all that understanding. While we're on it, if your doctor is so smart, why hasn't he cured you? And why do you suspect that he suspects you're faking your urine tests (damn it, you're not!)? And if he's so damned smart, how come he doesn't understand that you feel scared, even though you don't spell it out, and you feel angry.

Whew! Well, if it helps at all, you're not alone in feeling this fury. Not a person in the world who has diabetes doesn't feel like kicking it in the pants. Most of the time, you can control your anger or sublimate it into stuff that takes your mind off the disease. But sometimes, you just have a crawful. You feel resentful. You feel as though you could cry—the last thing in the world you want to do. And you feel as if you want to hurt back: punish THEM, EVERYONE, by not doing your tests, maybe, or not taking your insulin, by not answering to anyone or any damn disease! I mean, that's anger.

But deep inside you know that letting your fury out at parents, friends, doctors, siblings may feel good, may even be justified, but it doesn't really work as a general panacea. First of all, it makes you pretty unpopular and you hate seeing them hate seeing you, if you're really honest about it. Second of all, you don't seem to ever get anywhere with all that anger—it doesn't really work for you, and, in fact, it makes your disease worse. When your anger lingers on and on for long periods of time, you find your blood sugar rising, and when something angers you suddenly, you find you have an insulin reaction from a lowered sugar. It seems you can't win.

So . . . smart money says you find some magic to dissipate your anger, get rid of it in ways that won't make you feel sick or stupid for hurting yourself. Directing your anger at others, too often, doesn't get rid of it because it bounces back in the form of their hostility or hurt at being attacked. And like a Ping-Pong tournament, your anger keeps accelerating as it's propelled back and forth.

There are ways to soften a "mad" or a hurt and sometimes even get rid of it completely—depending on how mad you actually are. And these ways won't hurt you, a nice bonus. Try one on for size next time you feel your fists clenching . . .

Pound Something Many people feel that hard physical exercise that doesn't require thought is a marvelous anger-eraser. Remember, of course, to take the extra carbohydrates you'll need before plunging into an inspired jog, a wood-chopping session, a tennis game, an impassioned swim, a box-ing-bag pounding. Even if you didn't feel like expending the effort, at first, the mindless exertion and the sweat work-up are a real relief of teeth-clenching anger.

Word Smoothers Nothing smooths anger better than a frank talk with an unaggravating person. Mouth energy dissipates anger better than tranquilizers, every time. Ever wonder why so many psychiatrists get rich? Talking works! And you don't need to talk with someone who went to medical school. Your best friend will do just fine.

Mind Balms Meditation, TM, yoga, etc. Many people swear by the various methods of mind relaxation used for centuries by Eastern wise men. They require practice before you get the mad-on, so take a short course or read a few books on the various meditative techniques. Then, when you next feel your bile rising, go into your mantra!

The Pen Is Mightier Than the Valium It really is. Keeping a diary is not just for kids. The most intelligent shakers and movers in this world know the value of putting down your aggressions on paper. Somehow, as the words ease out of the pen onto the paper, they take the hurt with them. Someday, perhaps, you can even make a whole lot of money publishing your written anger. If there was *Diary of a Mad Housewife,* why not *Diary of a Mad Diabetic*—has a nice ring, don't you think?

Harness That Mad Sometimes, instead of yelling and screaming, you can harness anger and use it creatively. Much of the world's good comes from somebody else's anger. Start an organization of young people who need to talk about their anger and diabetes; compose a symphony, paint a picture. Use your anger as energy: write an angry letter, make a fantastic curry. Shape your anger and direct it to a place where its force can be used.

Open the Valve   The tear-duct valve, that is. Sometimes a good cry is absolutely satisfying; nothing else can beat it. You're allowed. And our society, that says men are weak if they cry, is wrong, wrong, wrong. Men are smart if they can vent their feelings in a good cry every now and then. It's like letting steam out through a pressure valve. Crying is finest when it's done behind a closed door or in a shower or somewhere else private. Then you can have a good, messy cry . . . the best!

THE TOUGH QUESTIONS

When you're an adolescent with diabetes there are a million questions you may have that your doctor or your parents try hard to answer, but somehow they just never seem to get it right. That's because there are no easy answers to your questions; and because the diabetes differs so much from adolescent to adolescent, the answers may also vary. The best way to get some satisfying answers is to sit around with a bunch of people your own age and see how *they* manage the situations that are currently griping you. We've isolated some of the questions from such group sessions held by members of the Association of Insulin-Dependent Diabetics (AIDD) of the Juvenile Diabetes Foundation, and we give you some of the solutions offered. They may be just what you're looking for; then again, they may not ring true at all. So use this section like a smorgasbord meal: swallow only what seems to fit your tastes, digest and use what is palatable, and ignore the rest. It takes a lot of experimenting and rejecting to get your act together.

Do I tell people about my diabetes?

Only if you want to. Many young people seem to feel that it makes them crazy to have to worry about keeping secrets on top of everything else. People think you're aloof and hiding something when you don't explain where it is you go every day (when you have to eat a snack, take a shot, test yourself, etc.). Further, keeping diabetes a secret tends to make it seem much worse that it really is—even to yourself. Many teenagers also feel more secure knowing that their friends know what to do for an insulin reaction. But, being fair, there are plenty of kids who feel that the disease is their own business and they prefer not to have people question them or to let it be known they have anything that makes them different from everybody else.

If you feel that diabetes is embarrassing or that it is a tremendous handicap, if you feel that it will somehow make you less attractive to other young men and women, naturally you're not about to spill the beans. If you want some advice (which you don't, but you're going to get it anyway), perhaps you ought to really dig deep inside to find out *why* you think having diabetes makes you unattractive. I mean, does it really? Does it make you ugly, clumsy, dumb? Of course not. If someone told you she had to wear a brace to help her walk or take medicine to help her breathe, would you think she was odd, peculiar, or a jerk? Well, if you would, you're odd, peculiar, and a jerk. The bummer of deciding to tell people about the disease, it's true, is having to educate them. You've got to explain what it is, and why you can do anything anyone else can do if your diabetes is under control. Having to do all that explaining—even though you give them the speedy version—can be a pain. On the other hand, once it's over, you're free! No hiding the testing, the shots, the snacks, and that's a huge relief.

The experience of many teenagers is that once their friends know, they totally accept it and pay no attention whatever to what you might consider your great "difference." The great difference, to others, turns out to be little more than wearing glasses. Anyway, do what seems comfortable to you. If you're happier with the secrecy—it's your secret. Perhaps, little by little, you'll come to share it with those you trust. But nowhere is it written that you have to tell or not tell. It's your decision to make.

Can I go on a weight-losing diet with diabetes?

Depends upon your age; and if you're still growing, you have to be very careful that the diet you choose has enough protein, which is needed for growth. Be wary, especially, about the big-name diets that have become so popular. The Pritikin diet, for instance, has far too little protein for an adolescent with diabetes. The *minimum* amount of protein you need, says Dr. Fredda Ginsberg-Fellner, is a ½ gram per pound, which means 60 grams a day if you weigh 120 pounds—and that's the absolute minimum.

A very good all-around diet is the Weight-Watcher's diet, which is sensible, providing about 1200 calories daily along with reasonable carbohydrates, fats, and proteins. Weight-Watchers even prescribes extra milk for growing teens. Naturally, be careful, says Dr. Ginsberg-Fellner, that if you lose weight, your insulin is carefully matched to the weight loss—otherwise, expect reactions. A general rule of thumb for losing weight is to do lots of blood sugars daily to make sure you don't have too much sugar; reduce insulin *slowly,* if that's necessary, and keep the protein intake at a reasonable level. But check with a doctor or nutritionist about any diet (including a vegetarian one) that you're considering *before* you go on it.

My insulin needs seem to be going bananas. What's happening?

Two things. You're growing, which means you need more calories . . . thus more insulin. Also, your endocrine activity is higher now and different hormones are being poured into your blood. They seem to inhibit the effectiveness of insulin, and so you need more insulin for that, too.

I'm a girl, and I seem to be having more problems than my friend who is a boy and a diabetic. Am I crazy or imagining it?

Not at all. According to Dr. Fredda Ginsberg-Fellner, girls *do* have more aggravation with diabetes during their adolescence. First of all, the estrogen sex hormones begin rising in the young female way before (sometimes two years or more) she actually gets her period, and that creates differing insulin needs that may change not only from month to month but from day to day. When the estrogens are high, she needs more insulin, and when they're low, she needs less. It's a cyclical thing, and since there's no test to tell you what your estrogen level is, this is a very tough time to maintain control. In addition to normal premenstrual tension, the increased need for insulin before your period and possible high blood sugar, anyway, will make you feel extra blah.

Don't be alarmed if you seem to have more than your share of abdominal pain before and during your period. It seems to be par for the course and is nothing unusual. The rise and fall of insulin needs around the time of your menstrual period may continue until menopause. What's the worst time? The year just before the first period of the menarche is full of emotional ups and downs and physical changes. Expect it. "You just have to resign yourself," says Dr. Fredda Ginsberg-Fellner, "to taking more tests and to adjusting insulin. Understand that your control will *not* be perfect no matter how conscientious you are." Teen-aged guys have it made in the shade when it comes to comparing effects of hormonal changes with female diabetic adolescence.

Will diabetes affect my growth, my skin, or my physical appearance?

If you are in control, it should not. Dr. Robert Kaye, chief of Pediatrics at Hahnemann Hospital in Philadelphia and one of the most famed experts in diabetes management in the country, says that there is no reason why growth should be affected *at all,* given good control—despite the fact that you see some very short adolescents with diabetes who have had problems with sugar control. You may have a zit or two or three, but don't blame it on your diabetes; blame it on your "teenness." If you find that you're seeing bumps or thickening of the skin around the injection area, change the site of the injections more regularly. There's an awful lot of space on the tummy that's no more sensitive than any other space and too many people ignore it. Actually, the stomach area is a fine place for injections because if you use it almost exclusively, the insulin in your body will always be absorbed at the same rate of speed. Using arms and legs, which are subject to different rates of exercising, tends to change the rate of absorption every day. It may be that as you are noticing such indentations, you feel as if you're actually beginning to dent like a fender. Here's a great tip: many JDF insulin users swear that the moment they stopped refrigerating their insulin (you don't have to, you know), the denting stopped and the hollow spaces filled in.

Another point to think about in terms of physical appearance: feet seem to heal slowly for anyone, not just diabetics. Try not to walk barefoot so as to avoid long-lasting scars from any bruises, cuts, or infections you may pick up.

> *I hate messing around with urine. What else can I do to check my sugar?*

It's a perfect time to start blood testing at home, a far superior method to urine testing anyway. You are not alone in your feelings. Many adolescents, particularly girls during their periods, would love to leave the urine where it belongs—in the toilet.

> *I feel so depressed all the time—and I just can't shake it. Is there anything I can do about it?*

Famed diabetes expert Dr. Priscilla White, of the Joslin Clinic in Boston, says that depression is found in all ages of diabetes and that does not exclude the teenager. If you feel sad—no matter how well you're doing at school—if you feel lonely and generally unhappy—no matter how many friends you have—it's a good idea to go for professional counseling. The Juvenile Diabetes Foundation can point you in the direction of psychologists and psychiatrists who are especially skilled at working with adolescents who have diabetes. It's not a weakness, it's a strength to know enough to ask for help.

Will my sexual function be affected by diabetes?

Probably not, if you keep your diabetes in control. Your sex life should be as active and fulfilling as your emotional state allows it to be. There is some evidence that some men who have had diabetes for many years develop impotence later in life, but there are also men who have had diabetes for over fifty years and never had a sexual problem. More on this in Chapter 4.

I'm sleeping overnight at my friend's and I just don't feel like hassling with the morning injection until I get home. Is that okay?

No, dummy, it's not okay unless you love feeling lousy. Considering the fact that you don't have to refrigerate the insulin, you can throw away all the equipment if you use the disposable kind; your friend has a bathroom where you can, if you wish, do the whole thing in total privacy. There's no reason at all to postpone that morning shot.

Can I postpone a meal if I have a sleep-over date and the family doesn't eat for two hours after my usual breakfast?

You do have a little leeway here, even though the rule is that you must eat to cover all injected insulin. If for some reason you must delay a meal for one or two hours, says Dr. Judith Wylie-Rosett, a nutritionist at the Diabetes Research and Training Center at the Albert Einstein College of Medicine in New York, eat a small portion of the meal like the bread at your usual mealtime, then have the rest later, when the family wakes up. Either bring your own emergency bagel or raid your friend's fridge for his bread—but eat *something* when you should.

My menstrual cramps are miserable and I was told that I shouldn't use certain medications (like birth control pills) to ease them because they raise blood sugar. What can I use?

Ask your doctor about aspirin or Motrin. These are drugs that inhibit the body's ability to initiate uterine contractions (as occur during labor), which are similar to menstrual cramps.

Who's responsible for my diabetes?

If anyone knew for sure, he'd be in Sweden accepting a Nobel prize from a grateful committee. Various theories abound, ranging from one which says it's the product of a genetic inheritance to the newest which says that a virus as common as the mumps could have brought it on. One thing's for sure: you can tell your ten-year-old brother who wished something terrible would happen to you in your last fight that he did *not* cause your illness. The guilt that others feel because of us doesn't help us one bit. My own father, a maturity-onset diabetic, once announced to me that he'd caused Larry's, his grandson's, condition. No matter how I tried to reason with him, I suspect he carried the pain of that thought to his death. No one knows quite how you got your diabetes. It's no one's fault. It just happened, like freckles. If your mother or father or brother or grandparent feels guilty, tell them to drop the guilt. It's not merited and, what's more, it makes you crazy having to be a social worker and reassure them all the time.

Will I be able to marry and have children?

Sure can. There have been astounding new advances in the care of the pregnant diabetic woman. Her chances of having a healthy baby get better every day if she's careful. And if you are male, you will be able to father a healthy child. More on this in Chapter 4.

Will I be able to go to an out-of-town college?

Why not? You should, by the time you go to college, be absolutely responsible for your own care. Your local doctor can recommend a specialist in the college area to take over your medical care. You really ought to decide to open up to roommates, teachers, and other friends about your diabetes. You'll carry snacks to classes, just as you did in high school, and you'll keep food in your room so you can stick to your own rather than the school's dining room schedule. In most schools you can rent, inexpensively, a small fridge—great for the orange juice, fruit, etc., you'll want to have around.

Why am I a "brittle" diabetic?

There's a lot of controversy about that term. Traditionally, a brittle diabetic is one who feels fine one minute, and the next minute, he's in the throes of a terrible insulin reaction. Or, at other times, his blood sugar shoots to the sky for no seeming reason at all. Dr. Alan Rubin of the University of San Francisco Medical College says: "There's no such thing as a brittle diabetic. There's nothing inherently abnormal in any diabetic which makes control impossible. Rather, people live brittle lifestyles: they don't exercise, they eat badly and they test ineffectively. . . ."

If your blood sugar goes blooey for what seems like no reason too often, your schedule must be individually tailored by the best diabetes specialist in town. You *must* test with home blood glucose methods if you've been relying up to now on urine testing. And understand that your "unstable" diabetes may also be very much a result of adolescence and, if so, temporary. Two new innovations currently being tested *and* used that may bring great relief are the insulin pump, which provides continuous insulin infusion instead of injections, and the new purer insulins—even human insulins.

> *Even if I'm generally open about my diabetes, I find it very difficult to handle when out on a date. Do I have to tell? If I do decide to tell him/ her, how should I do it?*

This is a hard one because there are many pros and cons to telling someone on a first date or even in the first few days. The pros for telling seem to be that most people accept the news as casually as you give it and it takes the burden of "secret-keeping" off your back—always a pain. Also emotions, which often run high on social occasions, do affect your diabetes, and if your sugar is high, you may have to make many trips to the bathroom (though this rarely happens if you're in control). If you have a low blood sugar reaction, it's nice to know that your date won't get puzzled when you whip out the candy, or panicky if you get sweaty or whatever you do get in a beginning reaction. It's comforting, also, that he/she will know what to do in an emergency.

Another pro for telling is that since you really have to eat pretty much on time—and you may have to ask in a restaurant if there's sugar in specific food—it's helpful to have it all out in the open in advance. Sometimes, in a new dating situation, this provides great conversation to get over the "small talk" period; whether you know it or not, people *are* interested in how other people cope. And look at it this way: if your date is the kind of person who would throw up her/his hands and scream at the disclosure, he/she is a witless loser whom you don't need. You've been asked out for you—not because you're rich or famous (unless you're Brooke Shields or Matt Dillon), and the fact of your diabetes should make little or no difference at all to your date.

On the other hand, there are cons: we'd be lying or patronizing if we said it was easy. It's not easy for *anyone,* let alone someone who's fairly new at the dating game, to disclose a personal thing—even though the very act of disclosure often makes you more endearing, more interesting to others. And there may be some people who become fearful at illnesses of any sort, who can't handle differences because of their own insecurity. Telling those people *will* be a write-off of any future relationship, let alone the evening you're presently involved in. But, tough gazoobies on them; even if your date is the most gorgeous, most popular person in school, it's better to find out about shallowness and fearfulness now than later. If you can't stand someone and feel that you'll never want to go out with him/her again, some kids feel it's not worth the hassle to start explaining about diabetes. Just get through the evening, is their goal.

Assuming that you decide, though, that being a candid person is the best way to start any relationship, just how do you do it?

You do NOT say to a blind date: "Hi, nice to meet you, let's not have any sugar."

Nor do you make a big thing out of the telling, as in: "It's very urgent that I speak with you privately, Seymour."

Nor is it a big joke: "I'll give you three guesses to find out what disease I have, Miranda."

What you *do* do is play it cool.

When ordering in a restaurant, you might say: "I wonder if the Hawaiian chicken has sugar in it because that's taboo for me and my diabetes." When you open the subject up, he'll probably have a question or two about diabetes, and you're off and running. Or, you might say: "Before we go out to dinner, I have to shoot up. It's not what you think, Arnold. I hope you're not troubled by this but I have diabetes and taking insulin shots is a necessary part of the pain-in-the-neck routine I've got to follow." Chances are he/she won't be bothered at all by the disclosure but will be fascinated and want to watch you shoot up. Then you can explain as little or as much as you wish. Funny thing about self-disclosure: making yourself vulnerable by telling something about yourself renders you very appealing, very attractive. Not everyone can be self-disclosing, but *everyone* admires someone who is free enough to tell a hard thing about herself. It kind of gives him "permission" to tell a hard or secret thing back, eventually.

So, if you decide to tell a date, wait for an opportune time, don't make any big deal out of the telling, and forget about it after that. The more you do it, the easier it gets.

Can I drink, smoke, smoke pot, experiment with other stuff?

Let's deal first with drinking. It's not terrific for you—you knew it before you asked. Still, if you must, do it in moderation, please. Always eat when you drink (and count the calories of the alcohol also, because an ounce of whiskey has about 85 calories, and an 8 ounce beer over 100). It's a good idea to have someone with whom you're drinking know about your diabetes in case the warning signs of an impending insulin reaction are mistaken for drunkenness.

Stay away from the mixed drinks that are loaded with sugar. A little dry white wine is a good choice; but the best choice of all is club soda with ice in it (gives you the feeling of drinking with no carbohydrates). Liquors, cordials, and dessert wines (like sweet sherry or port) are to be avoided because of their sugar content. Don't forget to count orange and tomato juice as exchanges when you mix them with alcoholic drinks. Never more than two drinks even when eating (sugar-free mixers don't count).

Smoking?

Don't do it . . . just please don't do it. It tends to narrow small blood vessels as diabetes also tends to do, and the combination of the two spells trouble in terms of future complications. Diabetics whose control is not particularly good have less oxygen in their tissues than people without the disease, and smoking, as it raises the blood level of carbon monoxide, adds to the decreased-oxygen problem. A recent study done at the University Hospital of Copenhagen in Denmark showed that diabetic patients who smoked had an average 15 to 20 percent higher insulin requirement than non-smokers *and* a higher level of blood fats. The word is not yet even in in terms of all the long-term problems smoking can bring to people with diabetes, but every single expert says it has to be bad news. Don't start; and stop if you already do smoke.

Can I smoke pot?

You will surely hear arguments for and against from your peers and even from the experts, but rest assured that smoking pot is particularly crummy for anyone with diabetes. First of all, it can easily act as a cover-up for an insulin reaction that even you won't be able to recognize. Your sense of time is distorted and you may not remember that you need to eat when you do. People who smoke pot report a definite craving for sweets—not so wonderful for you. In fact, horrible. Since no one really yet knows what pot does to non-diabetics, let alone to diabetics, after long usage, smart money says you try to avoid it.

Other drugs?

No. Please. Today's teenagers are getting richer and many have been playing around with stuff like cocaine (a narcotic), which makes the blood sugar rise because it alters the way carbohydrates are absorbed in the bloodstream. Other drugs like amphetamines (uppers, speed, pep pills) also raise and lower blood sugar erratically.

If you *didn't* have diabetes, drugs are bad news—all that junk floating around in your great body. With diabetes, drugs are worse news—all that junk floating around in your great body (which needs a little extra consideration over other great bodies).

Can I get a driver's license?

Yes. All fifty states allow people with diabetes to drive if you can pass the state's driving test. Some of the states require a teenager with diabetes to get a doctor's report certifying that the driver's diabetes is in good control. Certain states may give you problems about special licenses to operate buses, trucks, or other commercial vehicles, and current federal regulations prohibit insulin-dependent diabetics from driving these vehicles between states (interstate). Naturally, you will never drive without having a quick sugar source available in case you feel a reaction coming on. NEVER drink when you drive or take tranquilizers or allergy pills that might make you sleepy. Diabetes is not nor should it ever be an excuse for causing an accident. One tip: you know that emotional stresses can do crazy things to your blood sugar. If you are under a huge strain or even very aggravated about the last parental blow-out, don't drive!

Cheating—Who, me?

What happens if you hedge on your urine test? You may be tempted to "create" a better result on a urine test than the one that is *your* result. And no wonder. With the doctor talking about "good tests" and "bad tests," you feel like a criminal if the result is not what he's looking for. And your parents—hanging on the results as if they were pure gold. It's not surprising that you've considered taking an extra dollop of insulin when the urine test is 4+, or drinking a lot of water to dilute that urine and so give a lesser sugar reading. But don't do it. You may be doing yourself irreparable harm if the doctor is prescribing on the basis of inaccurate test results.

It's dangerous and unrealistic for either you or the doctor to expect your urine to be sugar-free twenty-four hours a day. If you feel that your doctor or parents are too judgmental of your test results, it's time to sit down and have a long talk with them. But don't bite off your nose to spite your face, which is what's happening when you tamper with test results.

What do I do if I'm really not cheating and still my tests make my doctor suspicious?

Get another doctor. Any doctor worth his salt knows that an adolescent can be meticulous about diet, exercise, and insulin, and still show elevated blood sugar. All kinds of things can happen, including a resistance to certain types of insulin. So do not *ever* walk around on the defensive, trying to prove that you've been careful when you don't feel like proving anything—especially when it's the truth. If the doctor doesn't take you at your word, she has little understanding of the nature of diabetes.

What can I do if I really can't talk to my parents because of their anxiety and fear?

It happens often. This is the time when you should really build up a close one-to-one relationship with a specialist in diabetes. He knows most of the answers to your questions and he doesn't have the intense personal involvement that gets in the way, sometimes, of true communication. Also, there's nothing better than a group session with people your own age. Your local JDF chapter will refer you to the group (AIDD) specifically formed for this purpose.

What sports are open to me?

Just about every one, providing you're in control and you plan for surges of extra activity by being prepared with a carbohydrate source. Common sense tells you that perhaps you ought to avoid sports like auto racing, scuba diving, sky diving, or surfing unless you can do them with someone. An insulin reaction during these sports could be very dangerous.

Besides camp, are there any other summer teen programs that stress physical fitness even if you're diabetic?

Yes, there are super ones! To give one example, the Diabetes Education Center at the St. Louis Park Medical Center in Minneapolis, Minnesota, organizes summer wilderness programs for diabetic girls and boys, ages sixteen to nineteen. They include hiking among mountain peaks and sparkling lakes, backpacking excursions, canoeing trips. Check with your local JDF chapter to hear about other possibilities. As I said—you can do anything!

Incidentally, here are some waterproof, portable snacks to carry as precautions against insulin reactions, should they occur while camping out:

- cake icing in a tube
- foil packets of honey (available in many fast food restaurants)
- candy or dried fruit in a Ziploc sandwich bag
- individual cans of juice
- corn syrup or sugarwater in a plastic bottle
- Kool-Aid with double sugar in a plastic bottle.

Is exercise essential?

YES. If you exercise at least three times a week, says Dr. Fredda Ginsberg-Fellner, you'll be amazed at how much better your control is. Do anything as long as it makes you work: swimming is wonderful, jumping rope is good if you hate everything else.

Studies have shown that the more you exercise, the less insulin you need. What's more, fat levels in your blood also decrease with regular exercise. Do it! Get out there and *move!*

What about diet?

This is the biggie: you can read books, tomes, whole libraries on the subject of insulin-dependent diabetics and diet. You probably already have. Along with insulin and exercise, diet's the very cornerstone of diabetes management. You cannot keep your blood sugar under good control unless you pay attention to your diet.

But you don't have to be diet-crazy. Common sense is often just as essential in diet management as the hundreds of lists of food exchanges, guidelines, forbidden fruits.

For instance, consider your morale. It's bound to be very poor if you decide you can *never* eat the butterscotch twirl ice cream, the pumpkin pie at Thanksgiving. So what do you do? You eat them. Not together and not often, but total deprivation is as terrible as eating too much. How much is too much? A baked potato the size of a football is too much. You'll know when it's too much. Come on, don't kid yourself. Current medical practice focuses on the ideal concept as maintaining normal body weight, relying more on calorie control than on specific amounts of carbohydrates ingested. Food is broken down, in simplest terms, into three groups: carbohydrates (sugar and starches), proteins, and fats. Most foods are a combination of at least two of these and all foods contain calories.

What *exactly* is a calorie? It's a unit of measure—a certain quantity of food that's capable of producing a certain amount of energy. You need energy, like an engine needs fuel, to make you operative. If you are very active, you need more calories to provide energy to make you go. If you sit around reading all day, you need fewer calories. Here's the rub now: if you eat more calories than your body uses, the extra calories are stored in chunk, otherwise known as fatty tissues. If you eat fewer than your body uses in energy, you burn up some of your stored body fat and you lose weight.

What you eat affects your blood glucose. The amount of insulin you take is therefore predicated on your blood sugar and what you eat each day.

The funny thing is that a diabetic's diet should be a diet that is fine for anyone: it should and can have unlimited variations to accommodate personal taste (including eccentricities) and lifestyle. You can be Jewish, Italian, Greek, Japanese, whatever, and eat according to the finest traditions of your heritage—and *still* maintain a healthy diet that is just right for a diabetic.

But there's one complication to all this. There are about a million diet choices that different people, institutions, doctors tout. For instance, there's

—The HCF diet (high carbohydrate/high fiber) of Dr. James Anderson of the University of Kentucky

—The Eat 40–50 Grams of Complex Carbohydrates and No Refined Sugar diet of Dr. Stanley Mirsky of the Mount Sinai School of Medicine

—The Exchange List diet of the American Diabetes Association

—The Low Carbohydrate/High Protein diet used by many young "brittle" diabetics and recommended by Dr. Richard K. Bernstein in *Diabetes: The Glucograf Method for Normalizing Blood Sugar*

And so on. It's enough to make you crazy. Especially when you finally come to realize, as you should, that each diabetic's meal plan should be tailormade, specifically designed for him/her. You need help, you really do, in this area, even if you're used to doing much of your own self-care. And you need a nutritionist who is qualified, not just a person who has taken a few food courses and had a grandmother who was a diabetic.

How do you find one? Dr. Judith Wylie-Rosett, R.D., Ed. D., is a nutritionist at the Diabetes Research and Training Center of the Albert Einstein College of Medicine and Montefiore Hospital and Medical Center in New York. A specialist in diabetes, she suggests the following as criteria and route to a true expert in diet:

You should insist on a nutritionist who is a registered dietician (R.D.), which means that he/she must meet stringent requirements before hanging out a shingle. You can find one in any of these ways:

—Ask your doctor for recommendations

—Check your local Juvenile Diabetes Foundation chapter or even the American Heart Association chapter (good diets for diabetics are pretty similar to those recommended by the American Heart Association for its members)

—See if any hospital outpatient clinics in your area offer nutrition counseling for diabetics

—Look in the telephone book to see if your area has Dial-A-Dietician. This voluntary service of the American Dietetic Association provides callers with general nutrition information

—Call or write to government health agencies such as your county or state health department or the Nutrition Division of the Agriculture Extension Service (telephone numbers can be found in your local telephone white pages under "Government").

Dieticians differ in fees, usually charging from $25 to $60, and these fees are sometimes covered by insurance. Make sure that your dietician, once you find one, creates a diet tailormade for you according to a thorough consideration of your diabetes history, which is recorded. Also keep this in mind: most good nutritionists require that you've had a physical examination no more than two months prior to your visit because complications like high blood pressure or high cholesterol levels can affect the diet plan being arranged for you.

Although your nutritionist will create a diet plan that's just right for you, I'd like to offer some general, good-sense ideas about nutrition that have been culled from years of experience and speaking with people in the field. Because exchange lists can become terribly complicated and cause you to be overly concerned with calories and amounts, try to think of it this way: the best diet is a diet whose protein source is not heavily fatted meat and that is rich in fresh vegetables and fruits. Carbohydrates like bread, cereal, vegetables, and fruit are yes-yesses. Proteins like chicken, fish, and veal are yes-yesses. Fats like butter and proteins like steak with all that white, fatty marbling are no-no's. Gloppy, sweet desserts are absolute no-no's. Glutinous sauces are no-no's. Seasonings, rife with sugar, salts and other substances poisonous not only for diabetics but for everybody, are no-no's. We've about forgotten what pure, fresh food even tastes like. You can almost judge the goodness of the food by listening to the inner voice that says: "Hold on. That's not so terrific-looking for blood sugar." If you *think* it looks like it won't do anything at all for your general health, it probably won't.

Dr. Fredda Ginsberg-Fellner recommends a simple but reasonable approach. Each feeding should be high in protein, with a moderate amount of starch and, if possible, no concentrated sweets. Saturated fats should be definitely limited. Skim milk is better than whole milk; liquid cooking oil is better than butter; veal, chicken, and fish are better than marbled-with-fat steak. Three meals and three snacks a day, says Dr. Ginsberg-Fellner, seem to create fewer low blood sugar reactions and better control than any other diet plan.

Can you be a vegetarian and still be a diabetic?

Sure, says Dr. Wylie-Rosett. You can be a lot of things and still be a diabetic—healthfully and successfully.

If you decide to organize your meal plans according to the exchange lists, you can get those lists from your local JDF chapter. As you no doubt already know, exchange lists are a method of substitution or tradeoffs to add variety and spice to diets. They're groups of measured foods of the same value in different categories (milk, vegetables, fruit, bread, meat, fat), which can be substituted for each other. For instance, if you usually have an apple after lunch but you're sick to the gills of apples, you can exchange a half a mango, a quarter of a small canteloupe, or ten large cherries for that apple, and still end up with the approximate amount of calories, carbohydrates, fats, and so on. Low-fat meat exchanges for 1 ounce of chuck steak could be fried shrimp, a quarter of a cup of cottage cheese, or 1 ounce of leg of lamb. It's a good idea to be familiar with these exchanges even if you don't allow your sun to rise and set by them (a very neurotic way of life).

What about vitamins?

The final word's not yet in on vitamins, and nutritionists differ violently as to their efficacy. Dr. Fredda Ginsberg-Fellner of Mount Sinai has this to say:

> "There's so much that's unknown in the field of nutrition and diabetes, let alone in the field of vitamins, but we generally go by this: because the urine volumes in almost all of our diabetic patients are higher than normal, thus spilling much of their water-soluble vitamins and minerals, we feel that extra water-soluble vitamins like a Vitamin B and C complex should be taken. There's zero data on Vitamin E, although it seems to be useful with babies who are suffering from retrolentilfibroplasia. Be careful with Vitamins A, D, and E because they're fat-soluble and excess amounts are stored within the body and can create horrendous complications. Over 10,000 units of Vitamin A or 400 units of Vitamin D daily are excess. A reasonable thing to do is to take a multi-vitamin because they're easier to get than the B/C complex. If vitamins are not overdone, they can't hurt, and they may well be of value."

Advocates of the controversial Vitamin C (ascorbic acid) like Dr. Linus Pauling particularly recommend the efficacy of this source. Dr. Pauling refers to the work of Drs. J. F. Dice and C. W. Daniel of the Department of Biological Sciences at Stanford University in California. They conducted a small pilot study which indicated that Vitamin C "markedly reduced the insulin requirement of a juvenile-onset diabetic." But again, the evidence has to be judged carefully because no large-scale testing of Vitamin C and diabetes control has been conducted.

So, certainly, diet and perhaps vitamin supplements also play a large part in the control of blood sugar. The best attitude is reasonableness. Sure you have to be much more careful than that irritating neighbor of yours who glops down Milky Ways as if there was no tomorrow. Sure you'll have to learn how to order in a restaurant in order to maintain your blood sugar, and what's more, you'll have to learn how to *leave over* excess amounts (or take them home in doggie bags for the next day). But don't be the kind of person like my friend Charlotte who consults a list before she opens her mouth—ever; who talks endlessly about her martyrdom (nobody loves a martyr) because she deprives herself of every good thing to eat, all the time; who is a consummate bore because she's a diabetic woman, first, instead of being a woman who has diabetes. Strange thing to note: with all her diet mania, Charlotte's blood sugar remains very hard to keep in control. Perhaps the stress of being compulsive works harder against her than an occasional diet lapse.

One last word about diet. You may run into the type of person (or quasi-nutritionist) who tells you that if you'll only just try a diet of tofu/ alfalfa/aspirin/sheep's genitals/and God knows what else, you'll be able to cut out your insulin. Don't buy it (the advice or the sheep's genitals, etc.). It won't work; insulin-dependent diabetics will need insulin until a way is found to teach their bodies to manufacture it. And as Geraldine, Lily Tomlin's telephone operator character, says, "That's the truth."

QUICK TAKE

The wonderful world of advertising . . . not so wonderful. Watch out for ads that tout things like

- "100% natural cereal"
- "Jello—the 'light' dessert"
- "Shake and Bake Barbeque Chicken"
- "Gatorade"
- "Hawaiian Punch"
- and other attractive-sounding products.

The sugar content of these yummy, "natural," "light" foods that America says are perfect for her natural generation is not so perfect for her generation of diabetic users. For instance, a box of 100 percent natural Quaker Cereal contains 24 percent sugar, which is more than Sealtest chocolate ice cream (21.4 percent sugar), Cool Whip Topping (21 percent sugar), and almost *three times* the percentage of sugar in Coca-Cola (8.8 percent). Sugar is the hidden ingredient in surprising things like bouillon cubes, non-dairy creamers, and Jello (82.6 percent!). Always read the ingredients even if they're in small print.

See the chart on page 116 for some general tips on nutrition.

SUGAR SIBLINGS

What is it like to have a brother or a sister who is diabetic? Of course, there are the problems. Sometimes he's a pain in the neck. Because of him, you can't have candy in the cupboard. Because of him, your parents pay you less attention. Because of him, you feel unaccountable guilt for your own good health. Sometimes, you don't feel very loving toward your sibling who has diabetes.

But sometimes you do. In the wake of trouble shared comes courage, kindness, love.

This is what my son Allan wrote today about his brother Larry who has diabetes.

> My brother Larry has had a great impact on my life. The earliest incident I can remember happened on a cold January day. The older boys were sledding down a steep hill called the "Balkan Trail." I wanted to ride the hill but I was afraid. My brother took me to the top of the hill and said, "I'll be with you all the way." With this said, and holding the sled as if my life depended on it, I was pushed down the hill by my brother. After a scary ride to the bottom I realized my brother had not been behind me.
>
> Looking back on that first ride I now realize that my brother was with me, has always been behind me and I with him.
>
> When he goes to the doctor to have a checkup, I wait eagerly to hear how it went. When he gives himself a needle, I feel pain. When the prospect of my brother losing his eyesight loomed in the background, I cried.
>
> I don't know what's different about growing up with a diabetic for a brother; I've never thought of him as handicapped. To me he's just been my big brother. And from my brother I have learned love, consistency, strength, and perseverance. With these gifts I can tackle almost anything.
>
> To my brother,
> I love you,
> Allan

The last word in Sugar Teens ought to be from the teens. What

Nutrition Tips for Insulin-Dependent Diabetics *

	EATING TIMES	TYPE OF FOOD	COMMENTS/SOCIAL EATING/ETC.
Infants	Feedings tend to be frequent and small, which makes control possible without major consideration to feeding times. Infant can be gently awakened to keep feedings regular and to cover insulin action.	Human milk and infant formulas include an appropriate mixture of protein, fat, and carbohydrate with introduction of solids at six months of age; some adjustment of insulin dose and/or time may be required.	Blood sugar can be tested using a heel-prick if hypoglycemia is suspected or monitor is needed. Rapid growth results in a high caloric requirement for body size. Appetite is largely physiologically determined.
Young Children	Parents largely control mealtimes but refusal to eat can become an area of tension. Regularity of meals and a matter-of-fact approach may reduce potential conflicts over eating.	Children become influenced by commercials and peers; requests for foods with a high sugar content are common. Allowing limited choices such as type of cereal within acceptable limits as to sugar content may suffice.	Social factor begins to play a role in eating pattern and food rejection. Exercise begins to play a role in balancing insulin and diet. Less insulin or more food is needed with exercise. Dietary choices can be used to start self-care routines.
Adolescents and Young Adults	Lifestyle is likely to be erratic, with irregular eating times. Home self-blood testing and multiple injections of regular insulin for meals can make lifestyle more flexible.	Simple sugar intake is likely to increase. Blood testing and use of simple sugar with exercise to maintain normal blood sugar can reduce conflicts around food. Fat intake is likely to be high due to fast food consumption. Knowledge of calorie content and exchanges helpful.	Social life becomes extremely important and peers largely determine food pattern. Self-sufficiency in monitoring blood sugar can help improve the quality of food choices and lifestyle flexibility. Extra regular insulin can be used for unplanned meals or snacks.
Adults	Schedule is likely to become more routine with work and/or family responsibilities.	Weight gain is common and limiting fat intake becomes even more important.	Social occasions are more likely to be planned in advance, allowing for adjustment in insulin dose and/or time.

*Reprinted courtesy of Dr. Judith Wylie-Rosett, R.D., Ed.D.

follows are some letters that we've received from young people who heard we were writing a book and wanted to get in their two cents.

LETTERS FROM SUGAR TEENS

Dear Lee and Sherry,

On August 20, I will be fourteen: that means I've been a diabetic for nine years. I would have written to you sooner but I've been in Alaska for six weeks. We take family trips there but I want you to know that I took my last trip, last spring, alone. I've learned one main thing on trips: always be prepared for anything. My father has a ham radio he takes when we go away to remote places together in case he has to contact someone in case of emergency.

I do real fine, actually. The hardest thing about handling my diabetes is explaining to my friends and new family members about it. Quite often, after I do that, they'll treat me special and I don't appreciate people thinking I'm handicapped. I'm not. So I usually wait till I know someone real well to tell them about my disease. My greatest fear is that someday I may lose a limb or have a reaction in my car or in public. When I was eight I had a reaction in a K-Mart store. All I remember is that people really stared.

I think that for every diabetic there should be someone who could be reached any time for advice. I find I can't talk to my family or my doctor; friends are a little easier, but sometimes I need to talk to someone who knows all about diabetes.

Tips I have for others? Only one thing. Don't consider it a handicap. Don't let it stop you from joining sports or taking trips. This is very important.

Love,
Christy Elizabeth Scott

* * *

Dear Lee and Sherry,

The hardest thing about handling diabetes in my thirteen years (I've had it since I was about six) are the sleep-over dates and the special attention I always needed, whether it was an extra snack, help with the amount of food I could eat, or shots. It's always a big hassle and everybody asks questions. I worry about if I'll have to run out of room to give myself shots. I worry about blindness.

I think camp has been my most wonderful thing. I don't have to plan for snacks—they're already planned and everyone understands. You don't feel different when you need a shot or a snack because everyone needs them and they understand.

I think people should realize that diabetics have to keep it in control but that won't stop them from being a success at what they want to be.

Sincerely,
Marguerite Madden

* * *

Dear Lee and Sherry,

I'm fourteen and have recently gone on the insulin pump. It's made a big difference in my blood sugars and in my personal life. I have more freedom to be myself and I feel a whole lot better, physically.

The hardest thing about handling diabetes is the misconceptions people have. They get all upset if they see you eating ketchup and then you have to explain the disease for half an hour.

With the insulin pump, here are some tips I find helpful: if you bend the needle at a 70-degree angle, it makes it much easier to tape down and it does not stop the flow of insulin. If I want to hide the pump, I wear a loose smock or flowy blouse. If anyone tries to take away the pump I'm going to put up a BIG fight.

I think I've come to terms with a big problem: my mom would constantly ask me what my blood sugars were and I used to think she was pestering me because she didn't think I could take care of my diabetes. Now I say to myself that she just cares and worries a lot about me and I try to understand.

Sincerely,
Joanne Moore

* * *

Dear Lee and Sherry,

What gripes me is the people who say you can lead a normal life. That's a lot of B.S. (blood sugar or whatever else you want to fill in). I've had this thing since I was twelve—I'm seventeen now—and there's no way anyone's going to tell me that sticking your arm with a needle every day is normal. Do I tell people? You better believe it. I look healthier and feel, in many ways, stronger and healthier than my friends because I take damned good care of myself. I have a reason for it: when that cure comes I want my body to be ready for it. And if it doesn't come? I expect to live my life, do everything I want to do, which includes getting married, having children, and maybe even running for Congress. Diabetes will not stop me from knocking the world on its ass.

Stan Solomon

* * *

Dear Lee and Sherry,

I'm sixteen, have had this disease for ten years and I still hate it. I'll never get used to it. Since I was twelve, and my neighbor wouldn't let her precious son swim in the same pool as me because she was afraid the kid would catch my diabetes, I've never willingly told anyone. I've also never been on a date. How could I? What would happen if I started to say weird things or act funny because of a reaction? Tell me, if you can, how to handle that kind of thing. You know what? You can't tell me a thing. There's no way of handling that kind of embarrassment.

Melanie Rosskeit

* * *

Dear Lee and Sherry,

My name is Lisa Pappas, I am thirteen years old, and I tell everyone I have diabetes because if they don't like it they don't have to be my friend.

Thank you,
Lisa Pappas

* * *

Dear Lee and Sherry,

I'm eighteen and this is what I have to say:

—On job applications, write "None" when they ask if you have any special health considerations. If you write that you have diabetes but it's well controlled, forget it.

—Work harder to keep up the image of a healthy diabetic. Even if you really are healthy you have to constantly prove it. The minute you're absent from school three times in a row, everyone assumes it's because of the diabetes and not because of the flu that has knocked everyone else out.

—First dates and casual acquaintances don't have to know your life story but you're kidding yourself if you don't tell people you care about. I have always been greatly surprised at how matter of factly my friends and even my girlfriends take the news of my diabetes: yeah? Well what else is new? Depends on how *you* view it, I guess.

—It's a lousy disease but there are worse.

Barry Cunningham

* * *

Dear Lee and Sherry,

It gets better, it really does, as you get older. I remember my mother crying, crying, crying. When I think of it now, I guess I'd do the same thing if I had to hold down a child of mine to puncture her arm.

What's helped me the most has been the library. I've learned things about how to handle my disease and what's new in the field that my doctors even didn't know. The next, most helpful thing, has been the Diabetes group I belong to. You can talk better to someone whose been there than you can talk to any doctor or even loved one. I resent having this disease, I think it's crummy that I have all these God-awful routines and worries dumped on me *besides* the usual problems of a teenager trying to grope her way to adulthood. I think sometimes it will turn off men who may become serious about me, although I don't seem to have any trouble with boyfriends and friends—and everyone knows. I make sure of that—eventually. If they can't take diabetes, I can't take them.

Basically, I feel pretty optimistic. I like me—even though the diabetes is the pits.

Let me end with a kind of peculiar thing I do that helps me over the worst times. I *reward* myself a lot for having to put up with all the junk. I'll buy myself more clothes than my friend buys *herself*, because she can eat the Hershey bar and go out for the beer and I can't. I'll indulge in more trips and vacations if I possibly can. Because I like myself, I think I'm allowed to make amends in some small ways for this pain-in-the-neck disease. It makes me feel less *deprived*.

Best.
Natalie Gross (seventeen)

4 SUGAR GROWN-UPS

The young, beautiful woman looked straight at her lunch companion and said above the restaurant din, "I'm going to shoot up now, I have to. I hope you don't mind."

"No, no, no," demurred the other woman. "Of course I don't." She really didn't. In point of fact, she was curious. She knew her friend was a diabetic but she'd never seen any real evidence of it. She was a little ashamed of being quite so curious.

The first woman took out a tiny syringe and injected it into an insulin bottle. "Bubbles." She shrugged with annoyance as she withdrew the needle from the insulin and tapped the syringe a few times. "There, that's got it."

With no embarrassment at all—at least, it looked as if she wasn't aware of the waitress and a few other diners staring with great interest—she reached down, hiked up her skirt a modest amount, and gave herself a life-saving shot of insulin right through her stocking into her thigh.

No one said a word. The diners went discreetly back to their hamburgers. The waitress smiled and set down the menus.

"The only time anyone ever said anything to me," said the young woman, who'd had diabetes since she was nine, "was when I did this whole thing in the ladies room. I was questioned, kind of suspiciously, then, but to do it openly . . . everyone accepts that you're not some kind of junkie. I've gotten used to it actually and I rarely explain to others what I'm doing. I don't feel as if I have to apologize or educate others every time I take a shot in public. If only taking the shots were all there was to having diabetes, it would be pretty easy. But there's more—a whole lot more, unfortunately."

She's right. There's a lot more to being a successful young adult who has diabetes than taking insulin shots.

Lydia Mann is twenty-two years old. She tells it as she sees it:

One of the least popular aspects of having a chronic disease is that there are no "easy parts" about it. When a person takes on the responsibility of shouldering a life-altering and debilitating disease, he gives up the option of ease. The old wives' tale goes on: "Saturday's child works for his living," and so "Diabetes' child works for his life."

When I had just turned nine, about Thanksgiving of 1970, I developed the first symptoms of juvenile diabetes mellitus: frequent urination, unquenchable thirst, lethargy, constant hunger. Within two days my parents had recognized the signs and had me in the office of a diabetologist (diabetes specialist). His attitude was "You're not sick. Thank God for insulin. Go home, call me tomorrow." I appreciated his hard-nosed attitude and stuck my chin high up in the air. My mother and I ate five dollars' worth of sugarless, Sorbitol-sweetened candy and suffered severe stomach disorders for two days afterward. We laughed it off and set about facing each traumatic change as it appeared: daily injections with the assistance of a Busher brand automatic injector, snacks, no candy, training up our friends and family as well as ourselves, and the innumerable subtle adjustments that occurred with varying degrees of success.

As I grew, I became more *superficially* responsible. My way of expressing this was hard cold toughness. There weren't tears or analyst's visits or any visible signs of weakness. I prided myself on being tough as nails and flexible as a palm tree. I would be responsible for all the trappings, inconveniences, and unexpected surprises of diabetes, but I would not become responsible for the integration of the disease into my developing personality. Over the years, I would take every intoxicant and drug and test my blood glucose in scientific experiments to make sure I would not send myself into diabetic shock or coma. But I would not confront the self-destructive tendencies that motivated me. I handled the body and not the self. I learned the medical jargon and maintained normal, on-diabetic readings on my AlCs (the blood test that gives a fairly accurate reading of diabetic control over a three-month period). I "did things my way."

And, like so many other diabetics, my body soon could no longer withstand the strain. Exhaustion, frequent minor illnesses, infections, and malaise had become my normal state of health. What's more, I was having great difficulty controlling my mind because I suffered enormous mood swings (probably in direct relation to my blood sugar swings), depression, and anxiety—common symptoms of poorly controlled diabetes.

Something had to change. It was me. So much new research points to tight control as a stopgap and preventative method for avoiding diabetic complications (blindness, kidney failure, circulatory disorders, etc.). There is no way to know how much damage I have already incurred. There are only processes left to change my course.

So I try. Diabetic diets are miserable. I tell myself, "You can do anything for a week—pretend it's just for one week." Each day I try to cajole myself into sticking to my 1300 prescribed daily calories, but I can't pretend enough. I know it's no week—it's my lifetime in this body and that's as good as forever. A "good" diabetic is the most disciplined person, and I am not. All I want is to be happy, and like a child enslaved by his senses, I don't always perceive my actions now as reactions later.

Polite folks say, "How do you do?" and I say, "Just fine, thanks," but what is fine? Is fine a 120mg./dl. blood sugar reading (non-diabetic range)? The calm of post–insulin reaction before your blood sugar goes soaring into the uncomfortable hyperglycemic stage? The peace of diabetic coma? The comfort of knowing your next injection or blood sugar test or doctor's ap-pointment or feeding isn't for a while?

A diabetic is never fine or normal except as far as the norm/constant is flux. A diabetic's condition is always volatile. Like I did (and sometimes still try to do), you can push the constant upheaval to the back of your mind and say, "That's just how it is," or you can try to grab hold of it and learn to guide it properly. Either way, you can never forget that you have diabetes, *are* diabetic. How can you be egocentric enough to take proper care of your condition? I, for one, don't think I could live with myself if I was. And who else will be? My husband? My children?

One way or the other, I combat a constant feeling of failure. Some-times I think it's a losing battle. Imagine Sisyphus and his boulder. Some-times I have high hopes. In the end, I think that we young diabetics must always be reevaluating our goals and setting them within our bounds. This is what all people must do to some degree. We just have more going against us than many others. And, ironically, since we are not physically deformed or bleeding or dying grotesquely and immediately, it is hard to realize the extent of our hardship. First, we must develop appropriate compassion for ourselves. The rest will follow.

Like Lydia, Adam Singer is also twenty-two years old. He is a gradu-ate of Wharton, co-chairman of the Association of Insulin-Dependent Diabetics, and a member of the Juvenile Diabetes Foundation board of governors. This is how he found out he'd have to live with diabetes and what he expects to do about the fight that's ahead.

I think I knew while I was driving to the doctor's office what the answer would be. When he told me that I had diabetes, all I could think of was "Bobby Clarke and shots."

There was no reason to expect illness. No one in my family had ever had diabetes, and I considered myself an active, healthy eighteen-year-old.

So why me? What was this illness and how would it change my life?

Experts now believe that diabetes is caused during a process by which a recessive trait is triggered by an environmental factor, probably a virus, that stifles insulin production by the pancreas. Insulin is needed to metabolize food intake in the form of blood glucose (sugar), so I must imperfectly substitute for my deficiency with two daily injections, attempting to control the characteristic swings in blood sugar, which can cause short-term and long-term debilitation.

There are so many variables to balance: insulin dosage, timing of meals, quantity and quality of meals, exercise, sleep, illness, for example. This is a disease that affects 2 million Americans. This is a disease that is the third leading cause of death in the United States and a primary factor in retinal, vascular, neural, and kidney system failures. This is a disease unanticipated by an optimistic teenager.

My mother was there in the waiting room, caring, waiting to see my reaction. Fine, a little numbed, thank you, but fine. I sleepwalked my way through the day, trying to call my father down in North Carolina on business. I needed to talk to him, but not to shock him. The feeling was more like bringing up a suddenly fascinating topic and wanting to hear someone else's perspective. The toughest moments were the answering silence on the phone when I reached him. After fifteen seconds I told him that I wasn't worried, so I didn't want him to be.

"Can't I worry a little?"

"Okay, a little."

When I tried to reach him an hour later, he'd already started the drive back up to New York. Actions say what words cannot.

The need to talk again. I sought out my friends and brother. Experiences had brought us to a point where we complemented each other like mind readers. I told them what I had, that I'd have to start shots, that I wasn't really worried.

"I know you can handle it, Ad."

"If you need me for anything, I'll be over."

Reinforcement: to know that I'd still be the same person, that others knew it too, and that they cared to treat me as before.

I didn't cry; the feeling was too new. After the novelty wore off, the tendency toward self-sympathy was short-lived. To use my illness as a tool or excuse was immediately repellent to me. Memory tells me that I took a walk and sat down in a field near my house to watch some kids playing baseball. I thought of my hopes for the future, for love, happiness, and success. I thought of a young child I knew who was seriously ill, and of the television shows I'd seen or articles I'd read on the courage of handicapped people. I thought of the courage and determination of a family friend, Jack Collins, who has been all of his life in a wheelchair.

Jack used to visit our house about once a year and I'd watch him and talk to him, fascinated all the time at his determination. Jack is considered one of, if not the, most brilliant chess mentors in history, his pupils including champions Bobby Fischer and William Lombardy. He has lived a life of challenge, of giving of himself to others, and I remain awestruck at even the hope of emulating him. There is no time to feel sorry for myself. Life is too precious and provides so much opportunity for the individual to act, to help himself and others, that for me to linger on my affliction would waste my energy.

I am actively seeking the cure for my diabetes. I've co-founded an education-intensive, peer support group, AIDD (Association of Insulin-Dependent Diabetics) which has expanded to more than twenty cities by mid-1982. We meet bi-monthly to learn from and support each other through our diabetic routines. As a volunteer for the Juvenile Diabetes Foundation, I am helping raise and direct money for diabetes research. For both of these groups, and for myself, I give speeches to doctors, students, businessmen, anyone who will listen and give me feedback and advice. I want to transfer the seriousness of the situation, while showing the hopes I have for the cure. I want to meet and share my experiences with other insulin-dependents, in the hope that our interaction may allow us new knowledge and a healthier life.

The future? I know that sometime in the next ten years I'll be "cured" through some medical treatment, probably the transplanting of insulin-producing cells. I'm confident I'll be in awe again, as I sink into pleasant complacency for about a week. Then I'll just have to find another problem to fight and cure, whether it's mine or someone else's. I'm hooked on a challenge; I hope I won't stop, because there's too much to do.

IT'S A TOUGH DISEASE—ALONE, IT'S UNBEARABLE. SHARING WITH OTHERS MAKES IT POSSIBLE

The name of the game is support. There ain't nothin' like it. When you're feeling down and low and you decide not to take your insulin twice that day or eat what you're supposed to eat, you *need* someone to say: "If you don't take your insulin and eat, I'll break your arm. I care about you. I know how you're feeling."

The Juvenile Diabetes Foundation has such a support group and it's called AIDD (Association of Insulin-Dependent Diabetics). Founded by Adam Singer of New York and Larry Ducat of Philadelphia, the group reaches out to others, and in particular to young adults who need to have *connections* with others who have diabetes.

This is a real account of a real evening. Many of the names have been changed to protect privacy, except that of Dr. David Mann, a clinical psychologist at the Albert Einstein Hospital in New York and a diabetic, who was invited to make comments and guide the evening's discussion.

The apartment was one of those chic New York City pads overlooking the lights of the skyscrapers, not to mention the East River. Low-dipping helicopters and sturdy tugboats chugging by made the whole thing seem like a movie set. Inside, the conversation wasn't quite so idyllic. It was with suicidal self-anger that the group of twelve diabetic young men and women were concerned on this particular evening. Only last week, one of its members had intentionally overdosed on drugs. She'd been found in time, but the news had left everyone badly shaken.

"I feel so guilty that I didn't hear what *must* have been hidden cries of help, hidden messages," said Lynn. "I can't believe that someone could sit here in this room, hurting so badly, and have no one know how desperately close to the edge she was."

"Well, I feel angry, if you must know," said Laura. "I mean, Bette was an important part of this group. She was a strong voice here. We need her. I think she had a responsibility to us also, not just to herself. It sounds cruel, I know, but I feel angry at her for trying to leave us, for copping out when we're all struggling with the same problems. She made me cry by doing what she did and the last thing I need in my life is more tears, damn it. She had no right . . ."

"It's clear Bette made an impact on your life and it's just a shame she didn't know it," said Dr. David Mann. "In a way, a suicide attempt is a way of throwing a tantrum for someone who doesn't know how to release her anger. She may have been feeling deprived. She may have felt she wanted to kill the illness—not really herself. Self-destruction can come from hating a part of yourself. Her feeling of hatred or deprivation may even have been coming from something quite separate from diabetes . . . and the diabetes anger just set it off."

"Yes, yes, I know that feeling," offered Carol. "Sometimes I feel that the urge to hurt myself is lurking in the background. I can handle it today but I'm not so sure about tomorrow. I wage a daily battle to control that feeling."

"Goddamn word—*control!*" exploded Bob. "A diabetic is constantly asked to test, test, test, to control, to CONTROL! Why should I have to control something I didn't ask for, something I didn't cause? And even if I do work on 'control,' there's no guarantee that my illness will be controlled. How do I control heredity, stress, luck—all those external factors? If my blood sugar goes out of control, I'm not a bad person, no matter how my doctor looks at me!"

"Right. That's where my anger comes from, I think," adds Maria. "I can be the best little girl in the world, do all the right things, and it still may not pay off. Yesterday I felt great. So today, I did the same things—took the same amount of insulin, ate the same foods, had the same exercise. But today, my blood sugar went up. So do I blame myself? Well, it happens, I do. I think I've failed. What did I do wrong? Somewhere, today, I didn't pass the test. I hate the doctor but I hate me more. It's terribly complicated. Somewhere down the line, it's my fault. Then I feel like getting back at myself for that—or at the world. You know how much time I spend thinking about my kidneys? I mean, no one should have to think about her own *kidneys*. I'm obsessed with my physiology—and I hate it. And I feel guilty when I'm not thinking about my body. Is that self-hatred?"

Dr. Mann smiles. He reaches out and touches Maria's hand.

"Just because you're not building up your body all the time and just because you don't do the right things all the time does not mean you're suicidal or even self-destructive. It's normal—even right—to get angry at doctors and even loved ones. If you think someone is doing a lousy job, like a doctor, even if he can't help it, you're right to blame him mentally. And right to talk about your pain. Rather than do a hurtful thing to yourself like eating the Nesselrode pie, *tell* someone you are really dying to eat it. That works almost as well. Then maybe you'll just need a bite of the pie. You'll do something *less* destructive if you share impulses with someone. And your anger may not last as long when you release it. Support groups are the best. There's no one else in this world who knows exactly how you feel except another diabetic. Only another diabetic understands your particular kind of fear."

"The fear gives me the most anger," says Sue. "If I had to choose between losing the illness and keeping the fear or keeping the illness and losing the fear, I'd choose to lose the fear. I think obsessively about going blind. Being dependent."

"Let me tell you how I've learned to help that," said Gary. "I research the thing that's scaring me. I read all about it, I ask a million questions. When I know all about it, what my chances really are of developing it, what the cures or non-cures are, what other people have done about it, then all of a sudden my fear seems to dissipate. I'm not saying that you should be morbid and look for things to go wrong, but somehow, if you're emotionally prepared for the worst, you have some readiness when a little hint of the worst comes. You don't waste your life worrying. You can't be surprise-attacked. That keeps me on an even keel."

"You mentioned about getting angry at the doctor," says Lynn to David Mann. "Well, yesterday my doctor said to me in an accusatory tone, 'That should have worked.' He was talking about something new we were trying. But it didn't work. And I KNOW he felt annoyed with me because his method didn't work. And I felt annoyed because I was so hopeful that it would work—and annoyed with *him* for seeming to blame me, somehow."

"But that's all right," says David. "That's being extra-punitive—if you feel you want to punish someone for failing you. It's when you become intra-punitive—you want to punish yourself for everything—that the trouble starts. That's what happened to Bette."

"I couldn't do without the group," says Lynda. "I have to tell you all that. It's a network of social support. Even if something gets you sad in the discussion, it's important that it come out. I felt like a marionette whose strings, whose *connection*, was cut when I didn't have the group to talk with. And that's all I want to say."

"Sure," adds David Mann. "If you go to strangers, even a therapist, and say, 'I am thinking about committing suicide,' those people outside your life can advise you, or not—they're still strangers. But if you come to me, a friend in the group, and you say, 'I want to kill myself,' and the friend says, 'What are you talking about, do you want to break my heart?' Well, that's somehow different."

And so the conversation went on. People who were not used to talking, to opening themselves up, seemed like experts at self-disclosure. There was not one person who didn't share. Who didn't feel somewhat more *relieved* than when he/she arrived for the meeting.

"This has been a heavy one," observed Maria. "At the next meeting, can we be a little lighter, please? Can we play?"

There was one observer at the group who did not have diabetes. It was Sherry, the co-author of this book. She had kind of an apology to make.

"When I asked if I could come to your meeting this evening," she said, "I was told that everyone generally brought something to eat. So I promptly ran out to buy a cake. Just before I came, I realized how thoughtless I was. And how it must happen to you a lot. And how difficult it must be to say No to desserts at dinner parties and stuff like that. So I put the cake in my fridge and I picked up some cheese and bread. And I want to tell you that I think my consciousness has been raised and I'll be more thoughtful of your problems next time I come."

"Was it chocolate?" asked Bob. "Did it have filling? Oh God, just tell me—was it *layered?*"

It isn't easy. But a little humor goes a long way.

AS THEY USED TO SAY—SHE HAS GOOD
HEALTH HABITS

It sounds like a cliché, but if you take good care of yourself in terms of personal hygiene, you have a much better chance of forestalling complications. Most of it, you already know. Here are some quick pointers on regular routines that should be part of your daily self-care pattern.

Teeth and Mouth   Diabetics are particularly susceptible to tooth and gum disease. An interesting aside: the fossilized teeth of most primitive men have been found to be flawless. Primitive men ate plenty of vegetables, whole grains, fish, fruit, and very, very few Good 'n Plenty's. You should be doing the same thing. Although primitive men didn't have Water Piks to stimulate their gums, you do: ask your dentist if you should use one.

To brush your teeth (at least twice daily) use a soft (never hard) multi-tufted nylon brush. Hold the toothbrush at a 45-degree angle to reach into the gum crevices (the junction between the tooth and the gum). The bristles should be pointing toward your nostrils. Vibrate the brush (don't scrub because that will injure sensitive gum tissues) for above five seconds; pull brush over tooth surface, sweeping away the plaque. First do the outside of every tooth in your mouth (when you do the outside of the bottom teeth, the bristles should be pointing to your chin, and then you sweep the brush *up* the tooth). Do the insides of the gums and teeth by holding the brush perpendicular to your teeth, fitting the top tip of bristles in the juncture between the gum and tooth (you really only need the top half of the toothbrush for this). Vibrate and sweep down (or up on the bottom teeth).

Brush your tongue every time you brush your teeth.

Floss in between the teeth and along the sides of each tooth, scraping away the plaque where the brush cannot reach.

DISGUSTING TIP: Think you don't need to floss? *Smell* the floss after it comes out of your mouth. Convincing? It should be! That's rotted material you're flossing out.

Periodontal Disease   In a long-term study, the National Institute of Dental Research discovered that children and adults with insulin-dependent diabetes have a far higher prevalence of gum loss and general periodontal breakdown than those without the disease. In fact, often the specialist in gum disease is the first one to suggest the possibility of diabetes. It's no surprise. The periodontal system is as much of an organ system as, say, the nerves or digestive system, and it reflects the body's health in the same manner.

Dr. Walter Cohen is the Dean and Professor of Periodontics at the University of Pennsylvania School of Dental Medicine in Philadelphia, Pennsylvania, and he says that a patient with a family history of diabetes, or one that is a diagnosed insulin-dependent diabetic ought to be aware of the following warning signs of periodontal problems:

- One or more loose teeth
- Bleeding gums
- Gum recession
- Spaces between the teeth you never noticed before
- Pus or other exudation coming from the gums or teeth
- A swelling in any area of the gum
- Anything that looks like an abscess on the gum

If you have any of these symptoms, see a periodontist immediately and make sure that the doctor understands the special problems that can come with diabetes. Dr. Cohen suggests that even if you have no signs of gum disease, you should be X-Rayed dentally once a year and examined at least twice a year. The periodontist should teach you how to brush, floss and otherwise care for your teeth and gums at home. He should show you how to use a "plaque disclosant" which temporarily stains the teeth with color to show you where plaque buildup has occurred.

An important suggestion: Dr. Cohen suggests that anyone with insulin-dependent diabetes be prophylactically treated (take an antibiotic like tetracycline) on the day before, the day of, and the day after a visit to the periodontist. This precaution will cut down on the risk of systemic infection during any oral manipulation—a real possibility for diabetics. Your dentist or physician should prescribe such an antibiotic.

Many people with diabetes have been advised by their physicians to use a combination of baking soda and hydrogen peroxide instead of toothpaste as a gum-disease preventative. Dr. Cohen says that in the four latest published studies on this procedure, all research has shown it to be ineffective.

What will the periodontist do? Gum infection is primarily a result of tartar (hardened plaque) on the teeth and in the gums. It has to be removed. Periodontists are wonderfully skilled at the deep cleansings that do the job. If the cleansing is not enough, you may need some surgery to get rid of the pockets or spaces of extra gum before bone damage occurs. If bone damage has already occurred, gum bone transplants are common practice; also, many modern periodontists can stimulate the regeneration of bone. But as with any other surgery, be sure you find a doctor who is experienced in treating diabetics. Large hospitals or your local Juvenile Diabetes Foundation can give you the names of such specialists. Try your dentist for a recommendation, also.

Bathing   The skin's the largest organ we have and it's essential that diabetics keep it healthy and free of infection. Bathing vigorously is great to stimulate circulation to the skin, but don't flay yourself with those loofah-type, abrasive torture cloths. Dr. Irving Abrahams, a dermatologist at Columbia-Presbyterian Hospital in New York, says: "Loofah sponges are supposed to take off the superficial keratin, which is the dead outer-skin area. I don't know why anyone would want to do that. That's the normal protective layer of the skin. It keeps the sun and soot off you."

Don't bathe in extremes of water temperature, either: boiling hot and ice cold are not particularly good for the health of the skin. Because hands carry much infection, wash them frequently; avoid chapping by using bland hand creams. Overexposure to the sun is not terrific for anyone, least of all diabetics. Use a sun screen and tan gradually.

Eyes   Since visual disturbances and even blindness are among the most feared complications of diabetes, it stands to reason that special care should be given to the eyes. Recent research has shown that good control is the most important way of preventing retinal disorders, so consistently good blood sugar is what you should aim for—I know, I know—easier said than done. But *try!* Diabetes is still a leading cause of blindness, but because of the new methods of home blood testing and of treatment, should eye problems show up, there's a good chance it won't happen to you. (More on eyes and eye care in the section on diabetic complications, Chapter 5, pp. 186–190.)

Feet   You want to be careful with your feet. Although the number of foot problems in diabetics is not significantly greater than in any other population, complications may arise more easily as a result of a decrease in blood supply due to arterial problems. Many diabetics also sustain peripheral nerve damage and then lose some sensation in the feet. This is a problem because when the normal pain sensation is missing, they can cause further damage by ignoring the trauma. Here are some general tips on foot care:

—Get in the habit, while you're young, of having your feet inspected at regular intervals by a physician or podiatrist who is quite familiar with the symptoms of diabetic complications. We've heard too many terrible stories of insulin-dependent diabetics who have gone to "foot doctors" for minor complaints; been cut and gouged by a foot practitioner who had little or no knowledge of diabetes; and have ended up with serious—very serious—problems.

—Inspect your own feet every day for signs of sores, redness, cracks or swelling in the skin, and any other irritations. For minor dryness and cracks, a quality emollient or skin cream should be used. Stay away from vaselines and ointments or greases, which stop up pores and add no moisture to the skin. Skin dryness is helped by soaking the feet in tepid water with a soft bath oil added, several times a day; dry until *almost* all the moisture is gone and then rub in skin cream. Between-the-toes moisture can be conducive to athlete's foot and other infections. Try cornstarch or a non-perfumed talcum powder, and if you suspect a fungal infection, see a doctor right away.

—Cut nails straight across, not in a V and never in the corners.

—Be very careful to pay attention to the corns and calluses that are caused by the buildup of hard skin at points where shoes exert pressure and friction. You can rub them down gently with a fine emory board or pumice stone; if they reappear, you should consult your podiatrist or physician.

—Walking is the best foot exercise.

—Most important of all, buy good shoes even if you have to spring for a few more dollars. Nothing, not fashion, not price, *nothing* is worth cramping your toes or impairing your circulation. If the shoe salesman says, "I'll just put them on the stretching machine for a few minutes," say thanks but no thanks.

One last bit of advice: buy only shoes of natural materials like leather. Shoes made of plastic or other man-made materials may be cheaper but they're hell on your feet because they do not "breathe," and heat and moisture are trapped inside the shoe. And think "low heels" if you're a woman.

—Socks and stockings: These can cause as many problems as poorly fitted shoes. There should always be some looseness at the toe to accommodate foot expansion when you put your whole weight down; socks should be clean; and they should preferably be of material that also "breathes." It's difficult to find "breathing" socks or stockings, so wear them as little as possible, opting instead for cotton panti-hose if you're a woman, and wool or cotton socks if you're a man.

—I know I sound like a broken record, but again, the best chance you have to avoid peripheral neuropathy (involvement of the nerves in the lower extremities) is to keep your blood sugar in good control, avoid smoking, and exercise daily. It's no guarantee that you'll be free of complications. Patients who have been *meticulous* about control also sometimes develop neuropathy; but you'll have a far better shot at a foot-problem-free life if you manage your diabetes routine successfully.

Finally, some don'ts from the U.S. Department of Health and Human Services:

- Don't apply hot water bottles, heating pads, or very hot water to your feet
- Don't wear cut-out shoes or sandals
- Don't apply strong antiseptics or chemicals to your feet.

Chuckling and touching Chuckling and touching? Yes, it's a very good health habit. There's little funny medical research to back it up, but there's no doubt at all in the minds of many doctors, researchers, and the "ordinary" people who have been the most valuable resource for this book that laughing, good humor, touching are therapeutic. Not just nice but healing and restorative. The social historian and author Norman Cousins wrote a whole book about his firm belief that laughing cured him from a dreaded disease. Laughing relaxes muscles, releases nervous energy and stress—something diabetics can do without nicely. Doctors at the University of Pennsylvania School of Medicine have found that touching changes heart rates and lowers blood pressure, as well as decreases pain. Hugging increases circulation.

I don't know how to tell you to get all this hugging and chuckling. Norman Cousins listened to funny re-runs of "Candid Camera" episodes that tickled his funnybone. One young diabetic woman we know simply announces to people, like her husband or her children or her friends: "Hey, listen, I absolutely NEED a squeeze, a touch this minute!" It works—for the squeezee and the squeezor also. What we're really trying to say is lighten up on your life a little, have fun, be silly, take vacations, prescribe some chuckles and touching for yourself, regularly. It's better than penicillin and *almost* as good as insulin.

Exercise

According to the *Joslin Clinic Diabetes Manual*, "exercise, whether at work or play, is as much a part of the treatment of diabetes as other forms of therapy. It is hard to overestimate its importance."

So whether you're a clod at heart or a jock, it makes no difference. If you're diabetic—you exercise. It doesn't have to be strenuous or violent but it should be consistent. And even if you tend toward the cloddishness, it really can be fun. You feel so *virtuous* after you exercise.

Why do you need it? For one thing, it tends to stabilize your blood sugar: not only do you have less high blood sugar but you also have fewer insulin reactions from low blood sugar, as well. And if you're a young adult worried about weight, you have to know that you can diet forever and you won't lose weight *and keep it off* unless you exercise. Jane Brody, writing in the *New York Times* about the newest "setpoint" weight reduction theory, says that "adding 200 calories worth of exercise to your day" is the best long-term approach to weight loss and maintenance. She quotes Dr. Martin Katahn, director of the Weight Management Program at Vanderbilt University, as saying that fat people should never go on a diet to lose weight unless they're willing to change their activity level. So there you have it: exercise is essential to maintain good blood sugar levels and to maintain terrific-looking bodies. You have no choice. You've got to do it. A few points to note:

—If you're over forty, get a stress test to see just what's the right amount of exercise for you.

—Establish your routine and your insulin intake accordingly, with your doctor. If you should exercise more than usual, one day, you *must* make compensations by either eating more or taking less insulin.

What follows is a table giving the approximate amount of calories expended in exercise so you can gauge yourself accordingly:

CALORIES EXPENDED PER HOUR	ACTIVITY
640	Walking (4 mph—that's a brisk pace)
720	Running (5.5 mph)
480	Ice or Roller Skating
600	Skiing
	Bicycling:
270	(5.5 mph)
660	(13.1 mph)
300	Golfing
600	Active Swimming
330	Dancing
440	Bowling

CALORIES EXPENDED PER HOUR	ACTIVITY
540	Football
470	Basketball
	Rowing:
740	22 strokes/min.
1140	33 strokes/min.
	Housekeeping:
190	Cleaning windows
280	Mopping
230	Scrubbing floors
780	Chopping wood

You'll be pleased to note, clods among you, that standing takes up 120 calories an hour and sitting takes up 108. If you write while you sit, add another 13 calories an hour.

One can benefit from exercise—it increases circulation, as you might have guessed, and that's good news for diabetics who need those blood vessels working at top level.

IF YOU DO GET SICK AND NEED MEDICATION, BE CAREFUL—IT MAY AFFECT YOUR BLOOD SUGAR

R. Keith Campbell, R.Ph., and Phillip D. Hansten, both Associate Professors of Clinical Pharmacology at the College of Pharmacy of Washington State University in Pullman, Washington, have compiled a list of commonly used drugs, what they're generally used for, and how they affect blood sugar. Before you take any drug at all, it's a good idea to check it against this list to see if it may have any effect on your blood glucose.

Commonly Used Drugs and Their Effects*

NOTE: The generic (general) name of a drug or class of drugs is given first, followed in parenthesis by one or more of the popular brand names. Drugs printed in italics can raise or lower blood sugar particularly severely. If you use diabetes pills, take special note of the drugs marked by an asterisk(*). When these drugs and diabetes pills are both used, the diabetes medicines can cause blood sugar to rise or fall even further. (Any time "diabetes pills" or "oral diabetes medicines" are mentioned here, they refer to drugs of the *sulfonylurea* type, the only kind sold in the United States.)

*Reprinted with permission from *Diabetes Forecast,* July/August 1982. Copyright © 1982 by the American Diabetes Association.

Drugs That Increase Blood Glucose

Corticosteroids (Prednisone, Decadron, Kenalog, Cortisone)* Most commonly used to relieve inflammation, redness, irritation, and swelling. Doctors prescribe corticosteroids for a variety of illnesses, including asthma, arthritis, multiple sclerosis, and myasthenia gravis.

Diazoxide (Hyperstat, Proglycem)* A powerful hyperglycemic (blood sugar–raising) agent used, under the name Proglycem, to treat low blood sugar caused by insulin-producing pancreatic tumors. Under the name Hyperstat, the drug is used to treat high blood pressure, but some doctors may not realize that it is the same drug as Proglycem.

*Diuretics** A broad class of drugs that relieves water buildup by increasing the amount of water passed through the urine. They are most often used to treat high blood pressure and congestive heart failure. The *thiazide diuretics* (Diuril, Hydrodiuril, Esidrix) generally have the strongest effect on blood sugar, but other kinds (including Diamox, Hygroton, Edecrin, and Lasix) can also raise blood sugar significantly.

Epinephrine, adrenaline (Adrenalin)* Often used as a life-saving drug to help start the heart after it has stopped beating. It is also used for treating asthma and allergic reactions (for example, to bee stings). Similar compounds are used as decongestants in cold remedies and as appetite suppressants in diet pills.

Estrogens, birth control pills (sold under several brand names) Used to prevent pregnancy and also to lessen the effects of menopause.

Lithium carbonate (Eskalith, Lithane) Used in treating manic-depressive illness.

Nicotinic acid, niacin In large doses, sometimes used to treat high cholesterol levels. Since it is a B vitamin, niacin is also sold over the counter as a nutrition supplement. Large doses can raise blood sugar.

*Phenobarbital** Used as a sedative or sleeping pill and sometimes for treating epilepsy. It raises blood sugar only in people who use diabetes pills.

Phenytoin (Dilantin)* Often used in treating epilepsy and other nervous system disorders. It does not raise blood sugar in all diabetics, but can have strong effects in some.

Propanolol (Inderal) In most diabetics, this drug *lowers* blood sugar (see below); but in a few people it can have the opposite effect.

Rifampin (Rifadin)* Used in treating tuberculosis. It raises blood sugar only in people who use diabetes pills, especially tolbutamide (Orinase).

Thyroid preparations, including desiccated thyroid Used by people who do not produce enough thyroid hormone or who have had their thyroid glands surgically removed.

Drugs That Decrease Blood Glucose

Anabolic steroids (Dianabol) Used for increasing muscle mass. Although seldom prescribed, they are sometimes misused by athletes.

Chloramphenicol (Chloromycetin)* A potent antibiotic used in treating serious infections, it has a number of side effects that limit its use. Lowers blood sugar only in people who use diabetes pills.

Coumarin anticoagulants (Dicumarol)* Used to thin the blood to prevent clotting, most often for heart attack patients. Lowers blood sugar only in people who use diabetes pills.

Fenfluramine (Pondimin) An appetite suppressant used for weight control in some people.

Methyldopa (Aldomet)* Used for treating high blood pressure. It lowers blood sugar only for people who use diabetes pills, particularly tolbutamide (Orinase).

Monoamine oxidase inhibitors, MAO inhibitors (Parnate, Nardil, Eutonyl)* Used to combat severe depression, though seldom prescribed because of many possible side effects. In addition to lowering blood sugar, they interact strongly with aged foods, including certain wines and cheeses.

Phenylbutazone (Butazolidin) An anti-inflammatory, used in treating arthritis. Lowers blood sugar only for people who use diabetes pills, particularly chlorpropamide (Diabinese).

Propanolol (Inderal) Used in treating angina (chest pain from heart ailments), unsteady heartbeats, and overactive thyroid glands. Not only can it lower blood sugar, but it can prevent the symptoms (including sweating and shakiness) that ordinarily let insulin users know their blood sugar is too low. Similar drugs are now being introduced in the United States (metoprolol, timolol) that appear to be safer for diabetics.

Sulfa drugs (Gantrisin, Septra, Bactrim)* Antibiotics, used for treating infections. They do not lower blood sugar on their own, but they are chemically similar to the sulfonylureas. When taken together with these oral diabetes medicines, they can cause a significant fall in blood sugar.

Over-the-Counter and Under-the-Table Drugs:

Like all prescription drugs, over-the-counter and "recreational" drugs can have unwanted effects, and they can sometimes interact with each other or prescription drugs. Because you can buy these drugs without a prescription, you must take extra care on your own to use them wisely.

Always read the label on packages of non-prescription drugs for general warnings and warnings for people with diabetes. But be aware that not all substances that can affect your blood sugar have warnings. The following are drugs that can affect blood sugar control.

Alcohol Alcohol can do different things to different people. Its main danger to diabetics is a severe, possibly fatal, fall in blood sugar levels when it is taken on an empty stomach. This tends to be worse in insulin-dependent diabetics and those who take oral diabetes medicine than in people whose diabetes is diet-controlled.

Ironically, alcohol can have exactly the opposite effect—that of increasing blood sugar—in individuals who drink large amounts over a long period of time. The increase is probably caused by liver damage.

Aspirin The amount of aspirin you would typically take for a headache or temporary fever is no great cause for concern. However, the amount you might take to control chronic pain may lower your blood sugar, especially if you take oral diabetes medicine. If you need a lot of aspirin, your doctor may have to adjust the dose of your diabetes medication.

Caffeine This is a stimulant found in coffee, tea, and many soft drinks. It is also the main ingredient of over-the-counter "pep" pills (Vivarin) and diuretics (Odrinil). Taken in large quantities, it can raise your blood sugar. Caffeine can also give you the "shakes" and may make you feel as if you are having an insulin reaction when you are not.

Cold remedies and diet pills Many of these medications—Sudafed, CoTylenol, Dexatrim, and Dietac among them—contain epinephrine-like compounds (including ephedrine, pseudoephedrine, phenylpropanolamine, phenylephedrine, and epinephrine). These substances can increase blood sugar (and also blood pressure) in some diabetics. The effect of these drugs also can make you feel as if you are having an insulin reaction when you are not. Never use any of them without first consulting your doctor.

Marijuana This "recreational" drug does not raise blood sugar directly, but does cause a craving for sweets in many of those who use it. Giving in to this craving can cause blood sugar to skyrocket.

Sugary medicines Most cough syrups and lozenges are almost entirely sugar. What's worse, they are often taken during an illness, when blood sugar tends to be high already.

Consult your doctor before using any medicine with sugar in it. If necessary, your pharmacist may be able to find a sugarless version of the medication you need. Many drugs are available in sugarless varieties, but be aware that drug manufacturers can add sugar to a product at any time without prior notice. If you are not sure about a drug's sugar content, write the manufacturer.

INSULIN-DEPENDENT DIABETICS . . . AND SEX

Admit it. If you're diabetic and over twelve, you've skipped over important stuff like traveling, nutrition, and job discrimination to get to these pages first. Let's face it: you need to know about everything, but there's no subject so vitally compelling to the average healthy adult as his or her own sexual prowess and possibilities.

What *does* it mean to be ripe for sensuality . . . and diabetic?

Let's begin with the women.

—Simply because no one else seems to much care. We've done a lot of poking around for this book, spoken to a whole lot of doctors, read other books on diabetes, and the usual response is an embarrassed "Uh, well, we don't know too much, actually," or a paragraph or so in a book. Perhaps that's because most researchers and physicians are male and the problem of female sexuality doesn't seem all that pressing.

Only three or four research studies of sexual response in diabetic women have ever been done at all and the results are very conflicting. Complaints from reputable sources seem to say that even these studies have been carried out under far less than perfectly controlled scientific situations. One study from Boston said that there was a somewhat lowered rate of orgasm in the diabetic woman. Dr. Robert C. Kolodny, director of the Endocrine Program at the Reproductive Biology Research Foundation in St. Louis, published a study in *Diabetes* (August 1971) indicating also that diabetic women reported fewer orgasms than non-diabetic women. On the other hand, Dr. Max Ellenberg, Clinical Professor of Medicine at Mount Sinai Hospital in New York and past president of the American Diabetes Association, indicated that his studies showed no difference at all in the sexual response of diabetic women as opposed to non-diabetic women, even when the diabetic woman had major physical problems like bladder dysfunction, ulcers, diarrhea, and other nasties—something that sounds just too unlikely to be true. How can you be sexually terrific when your stomach hurts? So there's disagreement even when there's any interest at all.

Dr. Arthur Krosnick, a diabetes specialist who is Clinical Associate Professor at Rutgers Medical School in New Jersey, says that's because, for one reason, the tools for measuring sexual response in women are just not very good. "Studies that try to draw conclusions from temperature measurement or vaginal tissue color are fraught with danger because the *normal* varies so much from woman to woman. And if the techniques are not great, by and large we have to rely on what patients tell us."

But that's not so accurate, either. What's terrific for one woman might be quite unsatisfactory for another. And Karen Berry, a sexuality education consultant and herself diabetic, brings up another point, what she calls the "stiff upper lip syndrome." "Women are often very slow to complain to their doctors that anything seems wrong," says Ms. Berry. "They act brave, stoical, develop an 'It's all-in-the-mind' attitude or 'Well, if my husband is satisfied, that's all that counts' way of life. I hate to sound defeatist, but how are we ever going to find out about diabetic women and sex if everyone keeps a stiff upper lip?"

She's right, and Dr. Krosnick agrees. "Never be philosophical and shrug off pain or an inability to have an orgasm," he says. "That can make life very unpleasant." Lynne Wabrek, the co-director of the Sexual Therapy Program at Hartford Hospital in Connecticut, adds that she's observed psychological problems with sexuality from what she terms "Stop-Start" effect. Many gynecologists too easily prescribe that their women patients "just abstain for a while" when they have minor infections, says Ms. Wabrek; this is hugely distracting to the female diabetic, who finds it difficult regularly to turn her sexual appetites on and off as she'd turn a water faucet.

So there *may* be real problems—not terribly dramatic because the female doesn't have to maintain an erection and can really always be physically available for intercourse, but pretty grim if one's enjoyment is hampered. The frustrating part about all this is that when and if problems arise, *they can often easily be solved* with just a little education, if only, say the concerned doctors and sex therapists, women were not too embarrassed to ask for help.

Take, for instance, one of the problems that seems to plague women who have had diabetes for a long time. A major sign of arousal in a female is the lubrication produced by her genitals during sex activity; in long-term diabetes, says Dr. Krosnick, small blood vessels in the skin and in the mucous membranes tend to get blocked off, thus hampering the secretion of vaginal fluids. This creates a drier vaginal condition, which tends to make intercourse not only uncomfortable but sometimes downright painful. There are things to do like using an ordinary, water-soluble surgical lubricant such as K-Y jelly, which helps the dryness and does not affect diabetes control at all. Regular petroleum jelly may inhibit your own natural secretions and is not advised. "If vaginal dryness is due to an estrogen deficiency, sometimes using an estrogen cream as infrequently as three times weekly can be very helpful, especially to the older woman," says Dr. Krosnick.

Another problem may arise from psychological pressures. Karen Berry of Connecticut says that her own studies of one hundred diabetic women show there may well be "mild arousal interference" in those women who are worried that they'll have an insulin reaction on top of an orgasm—making it quite difficult, to say the least, to relax and enjoy.

The best thing any woman can do for her own sexuality is to try to keep her blood sugar in control. This helps enormously. Assuming that blood sugar is in control, says Dr. Krosnick, apparently "the ability of diabetic women to reach orgasm does not appear to be hampered. The impression we've been getting is that the degree, quantity, and quality of their orgasms are probably normal or very close to it . . . even if they have some evidence of other diabetic neuropathy."

It makes sense. You only need sound reasoning, not doctors, to tell you that the better your diabetes is controlled, the more successful sexually you'll be. When your sugar is high, you feel crummy, tired, and not terribly romantic. When your urine sugar is high, it may affect the vaginal tissues, promoting the growth of yeast and bacteria, which, in turn, result in infections—swelling, itching, burning, the feeling you have to urinate incessantly. Even though drugs and salves can relieve infections, nothing is going to make you happily lusty until that diabetes is under control.

The bottom line is that if you take good care of keeping your blood sugar down, the picture looks quite good. But be aware that the final scientific word on just how diabetes affects you physically and emotionally in your sexuality is not yet in, despite the fact that most doctors and books written on diabetes say that women have nothing to worry about. Chances are, you'll be fine. But listen—if a problem crops up, ask questions! Don't let anyone tell you that any sexual discomfort should be ignored. Most major hospitals can guide you to a knowledgeable doctor or sexuality educator. If the women's movement has done anything at all for you, it should have led you at least to expect more than the mild statement on the subject that Dr. Milton Brothers (husband of Joyce) puts out. Speaking of the neuropathy that may indeed hamper sexual arousal in women, he says: "If one agrees, however, that women have a right to experience orgasm, and the time seems right to agree, it is indeed a distressing disorder." Don't wait for anyone to agree that you have a right to experience orgasm. Insist on your right.

And now to the men:

There are better techniques for measuring sexuality in diabetic men than in women. And although there are more demonstrable problems, there are also more possibilities available for recourse.

First of all, diabetes does not make you less interested in sex. It does not end your fertility or your capacity to ejaculate or have an orgasm. What it can do, to *some* men—certainly very far from all diabetic men—is to diminish and maybe even in more drastic cases eventually bring to an end the ability to have an erection. Sometimes the reasons for this are physical and sometimes they're psychological. But whatever the reason, whenever a man cannot have or maintain an erection, he's said to be impotent—and that, to put it as mildly, as politely as possible, is quite a drag. First, let's look at the most probable *physical* reasons why this can occur in a male diabetic:

1. He may have neuropathy (damaged nerves). When a man is sexually turned on, the pelvic nerves cause the arteries into the penis to expand. This allows the blood to rush in, and *voilà*—an erection. But when there is neuropathic damage to those pelvic nerves, they don't work so well, or sometimes, at all, and the man is not able to "start, sustain, and successfully complete the act of intercourse."

Estimates vary on how probable an occurrence this is with men who have diabetes. Although, again, it surely doesn't always happen. Dr. Steven Gabbe, Associate Professor of Obstetrics and Gynecology at the Hospital of the University of Pennsylvania in Philadelphia, says there is a higher frequency of impotence (about 50 percent higher) in males with diabetes than in males without diabetes, and this statistic is confirmed by researchers at the Jefferson Hospital in Philadelphia where ongoing studies on impotence are being carried out. When does it happen? Some studies have shown that by the time a diabetic male reaches fifty or sixty years of age, he has about a 50 percent chance of impotency; others have shown that nearly 30 percent of male diabetics under the age of thirty have some erectile disorders. But impotence is not inevitable. There's a reasonably good chance that a diabetic male will *not* become impotent, at least not as a result of his diabetes.

2. He may have a vascular condition like arteriosclerosis, which involves the thickening of vessel walls and therefore creates a lesser blood flow to the penis, making erection more difficult.

3. He may have poorly controlled blood sugar, which can cause malnutrition and general weakness, all of which don't do a whole lot for potency. There is much controversy about whether the quality of blood sugar control through the years really is a cause of physical impotence, but the most prominent doctors today seem to buy the theory that it is. There has also been a great deal of controversy on the issue of whether just older men who have had poorly controlled diabetes for a long while become most easily impotent—or whether younger men are also more susceptible than previously thought. Sometimes, whatever the age, a man can develop a temporary impotence that goes away when he's able to control his blood sugars more carefully.

There are *psychological* anxieties that can easily bring on impotence in men with diabetes. When a man reads that he may become impotent from his disease, when he hears that his best friend, also diabetic, has just gone through such a draining experience, he tends to carefully watch his own "performance," often worrying himself limp in more ways than one. The gurus of sexuality, Masters and Johnson, called this "spectatoring"; and Raul C. Schiavi and Barbara Hogan described it in an article for *Diabetes Care* this way: "The diabetic patient, rather than becoming involved in the sexual experience and abandoning himself into erotic sensations and feelings, may find himself constantly monitoring the state of his penis. He becomes a witness rather than a participant in the sexual experience." Not easy to be a star when you're a nervous observer.

Psychological impotence happens more frequently than you'd imagine with men who are *free* of chronic diseases. Imagine, then, the effect on a man who's got some clearer cause for concern . . . no matter how intellectually aware of the fact that it is far from a sure thing to happen.

If you're a male with diabetes and you're having some concerns about your sexuality, first find out if the reasons for your concern are physical or psychological. Although the two often overlap and it's not so clear-cut, there's one fascinating test that almost always proves it one way or another. If a visit to a diabetologist, neurologist, or urologist doesn't turn up any physical reasons for impotency, your doctor may suggest an NPT (Nocturnal Penile Tumescence) assessment. NPT refers to the erections that normally occur during one state of a man's sleep pattern—the rapid eye movement stage—usually the dreaming time. He can be getting glorious erections during this period and unfortunately not remember a thing about them in the morning. But if he's getting erections in sleep (and this test is usually done in the sleep laboratory of a medical center), his impotency is not caused by a physical problem. If the man is not having erections in his sleep at all, his impotency may be due to nerve damage.

Some other clues as to the physical versus the psychological reasons: if your impotency is caused by psychological anxiety, it may come on very suddenly, even overnight. When it's physically caused, it may take months, even years to develop. When the problem is caused by a physical reason, your libido, lust, desire—call it what you want—is usually always still very much there. When you have a psychological problem with maintaining an erection, often your true desire to have sexual relations is dulled by your fear that you won't be successful. You talk yourself out of wanting it so much, in essence. It's a terribly complicated business.

Okay: what can you do about it?

If the problem is psychological, you need to talk about it—to a person who knows something about diabetes and the anxiety it may incur. Just anyone who hangs out a shingle saying 'Sex Therapist' will not do. And even if you are treated by a reputable therapist recommended by your doctor or a major medical center, don't be disappointed if the whole thing doesn't immediately go away just because you intellectually understand what's happening. It's one thing for your head to know that fear is causing impotence; it's another thing for your groin to *believe* it. Be patient. Better days—and nights—lie ahead.

If the problem is physically caused, there are also remedies. If neuropathy is behind it, you have to understand that you can't (yet) fix damaged nerves. If a patient has total impotence, he may opt to try a surgical implant (after discussion, naturally, with his sex partner). Two kinds are available. One is an inflexible silicone prosthesis, which can be surgically implanted into the penis, creating a partial erection that will allow for penetration, ejaculation, and orgasm. The problem with this is that the implant is rigid and keeps the penis erect—all the time. It's not really visible, though, under clothing, because, as stated, it's not a full erection. The other possibility is more complicated but perhaps more natural, because it is an "inflatable erectile," also implanted into the penis, and this number can become rigid or relax as you wish.

Dr. Stanley Mirsky and Joan Rattner Heilman in their book *Diabetes: Controlling It the Easy Way* offer a very sensible suggestion. The partner of the man with neuropathy can learn to build up her vaginal muscles in order to be able to hold a "somewhat thinner" penis and make sexual activity more fulfilling for both. She can do an exercise called the Kegel Exercise, which consists of alternate tightening and releasing of the vaginal-rectal muscles for about ten minutes every day; another way of thinking of the Kegel Exercise is to imitate what it is you do when you have to urinate and there's no toilet for six blocks.

If impotency is caused by a vascular condition, a variety of new by-pass operations are being studied and some have proved wonderfully successful.

If the impotency is caused by poor blood sugar control, often the problem clears up just by better diabetes management.

You do know, also, that certain substances including marijuana, tranquilizers, and alcohol among others can cause temporary impotence (and all the while you were laying it on the diabetes!).

One more idea: Dr. Richard Bernstein in *Diabetes: The Glucograf Method for Normalizing Blood Sugar* says he feels that low blood glucose (hypoglycemia) can impair sexual functioning (and he's been a diabetic for many years). Indeed, says Dr. Bernstein, for insulin-dependent diabetics, it's probably the most common cause of sexual dysfunction. It's "an early warning sign that's been detected by both males and females. In fact, some patients have located the BGL's [blood glucose levels] at which they 'turn off.'" Dr. Bernstein adds that at a certain blood glucose level both men and women can be aroused but cannot achieve orgasm, and when the blood glucose is even lower, they cannot even be aroused.

So there you have it:

—If you're a male and diabetic, you may never in your life have a serious problem with impotency that's due to diabetes.

—If you do have impaired potency, there are new things to try and much that's currently being researched. Many of the doctors who are in diabetic research are themselves male and diabetic. That's a very good reason to suspect that new solutions are being considered.

Finally, if you are a young male adult reading this book and you suspect you may be having some difficulty with erections, don't wait for your doctor to open up the subject. He/she may be waiting for you to bring it up. Dr. Fredda Ginsberg-Fellner comments: "We never thought our very young male patients worried about this so much, but they do. They're no fools, they read, they hear, this current crop of kids. Many of them have

sexual relations very early because they want to know if they're all right—
they feel a time pressure. If they don't ask, we bring up the subject directly,
now. It's important to get the thing out of the closet. Young people in their
late teens and early twenties have had some partial problems even if that's
pretty rare. But since blood control is very important, it should be discussed
with your doctor."

Know one thing. Your macho qualities, your manhood, should never
be affected by any impotency episodes, even if that sounds like a Pollyanna-
ish statement. It is absolutely true. There are marvelous and sweet ways of
satisfying partners and yourself without intercourse—should you develop
an impotency problem. And it's possible to nurture relationships, even in
the face of such difficulty, that are stronger, dearer, and more significant
than was ever before possible for you—simply because of adversity shared.

CONTRACEPTION

First, the good news. Many things, including the famed Pill, IUDs (intra-
uterine devices), diaphragms, condoms, and contraceptive foams, work.
Some work a whole lot better than others.

Now, the bad news. If you have diabetes, you'd better be quite careful
about the method of contraception you choose. There are strong contra-
indications (reasons why you shouldn't do it) to using either the Pill or an
IUD. Diabetic women stand a higher risk of pregnancy-related problems
than non-diabetic women, so it's essential to find something you can trust.
Although diabetes surely limits our options, it doesn't close them off. Now
isn't that good news?

We went directly to the top to find out the pros and cons for this
book. Lin Campbell, an extraordinarily knowledgeable executive with
Planned Parenthood, is herself a diabetic woman who has had careless doctors prescribe birth control methods for her that would have likely created
disastrous complications—had she listened blindly. That's an experience
not unique among young diabetic women. Lin says: "In the end, taking care
of yourself is your own responsibility. Don't ever give it away to someone
who has a title but who may not know as much as you do about diabetes.
Planned parenthood, of course, depends on people selecting a method that
they'll use; it doesn't matter how effective a method is if you're not comfortable with it." Lin's suggestions, supported by many top gynecologists
and diabetes experts, follow.

The Combined Pill It's an orally taken, combined hormone (estrogen and progestogen) contraceptive, and it's used by millions of women

throughout the world. Theoretically, it's close to 100 percent effective. But there *are* cardiovascular problems associated with it and diabetic women on the Pill have a "considerably greater risk" of cardiovascular and cerebrovascular disease than non-diabetic women, according to studies reported in both the *Journal of the American Medical Association* and the *British Medical Journal* in 1975. When you take the Pill, a certain amount of vasoconstriction takes place, causing the user's arteries to thicken. This opens you up, particularly if you're a diabetic and prone to such problems, to a higher risk of blood clots or stroke. Certainly *anyone* with circulatory problems should not use the Pill. Furthermore, it elevates the vagina's body temperature, making it a more favorable environment for infection, and diabetic women who have anyway a higher risk of vaginal and urinal infections ought not to fool around with an increased risk of more problems.

Some studies have shown that hormones in the Pill can lower your glucose tolerance and, in turn, cause your insulin to be somewhat more ineffective. Thus, it appears that the Pill is far from your best choice. There *is* another kind of Pill—one that contains only progestin, which seems to be safer for diabetic women. Check with your doctor on pros and cons.

IUDs   A device that's fitted inside the uterus and theoretically about 95 to 98 percent effective. It's another poor choice for you. There are much higher risks than normal of pelvic infection, inflammatory disease, and other problems with IUDs than with condoms and foam contraceptives. According to a recent (March 1982) article in the British medical journal *The Lancet,* there's a 36 percent higher failure (pregnancy) rate in IUD users who are diabetic than in non-diabetic users. So, an IUD is pretty much out also, drat it.

The Diaphragm   It's a dome-shaped rubber cup with a flexible rim that's inserted into the vagina before intercourse, and used with a spermicidal agent inside the diaphragm for best results. Theoretically it's quite effective, but its effectiveness is dependent on proper use, which can be tricky because it has to be used at every intercourse, fitted properly, inserted properly, left in for at least six hours after intercourse. All of these "musts" make it *actually* less effective than the following method, which most doctors and experts in the field of diabetes like to recommend.

The Condom and Foam   The condom is a rubber or processed tissue sheath that fits over the man's erect penis and catches the semen before it can reach the vagina. It has no side effects unless you're allergic to the spermicidal agent that should be placed inside the condom for best results. Theoretically, the rate of safety of the condom, when used with foam, approaches that of the Pill; but actually it's lower because many users complain that it "feels like taking a shower with a raincoat on," or "shaking hands with gloves on." Too many "forget" to put it on at the crucial moment. Still others, particularly teenagers, don't like to have "evidence" around for their families to see—if they have a need for secrecy.

But because condoms used with foam (without foam, they're less safe) are the contraceptive of choice for people who are diabetic, a real effort ought to be made to give them a chance. Try the natural skin condoms if you feel that the less expensive ones are not sensitive enough. They are so thin they're hardly felt at all, and they're more reliable against breakage, leaking, and other nasties, even if they are more costly.

CAUTION: Don't be duped by misleading advertisements saying that *vaginal spermicides,* which are foaming agents used to kill the sperm, work as well as the Pill. They don't. Encare Ovals or Encare are foams and vaginal suppositories that are effective with condom use but whose effectiveness *alone* still needs corroboration. If you can stand the fizz (some people say it turns them on), use it in conjunction with a condom, but don't depend on it alone.

A Word About Insulin Pumps and Sex At this stage of the game, insulin pumps are somewhat bulky and not exactly erotic. Check with your physician, of course, but common sense dictates that there's no reason you can't take it off during love-making. Unless, of course, your partner is extremely weird and insulin pumps really turn him/her on.

IS MARRIAGE IN MY PICTURE?

People with diabetes have married people with or without diabetes and have been extraordinarily happy. They've built productive lives, had healthy families, been closer and in some cases more successful sexually and emotionally than their counterparts who have no illnesses more serious than colds. So, sure, marriage is in your picture if you find someone you'd like to marry.

Still, there are problems, no getting around it. The problems are not insurmountable if you both want each other enough and are willing to educate yourselves about what's involved in marrying diabetes. Because you're doing just that: along with the person you love, you're marrying his/her diabetes routine. Full knowledge of what that means ought to take place in many self-disclosing, absolutely honest conversations before your marriage. Here are some points that ought to be included in those conversations.

> *Can the presence of diabetes in a marriage bring more than the usual amount of emotional stress?*

Sure it can. Anyone who denies it is lying through their teeth. The divorce rate among diabetics is high. Diabetes (blood sugars high and low) can affect the disposition—you're grumpy and irritable if your blood sugar is high. Secret frustrations abound: sticking to a diet when the rest of the family is wolfing down sundaes; baking for a family only to watch them happily consume the product while you practice restraint; having to stick to rigid time schedules for eating and exercise; being responsible for great expenses in the family not only to maintain proper control but in terms of emergencies, pregnancies, surgeries; living with the possibility of complications no matter how careful and "good" you are; living with the special problems of insurance, employment, insulin reactions. They *all* cause emotional ups and downs. Which doesn't mean you ought to decide against marriage; it just means that before the marriage, a lot of good, honest talk should go on and all of these possibilities should be considered.

Can you deal with the emotional stresses that a chronic illness can bring? If you think you can, you probably can. Having diabetes as a bedfellow doesn't automatically bring trouble between you. Just consider that the national divorce rate is one out of every two marriages and most of these have nothing to do with blood sugar. One thing's for sure: in a marriage where one spouse uses diabetes as an excuse for acting unfairly, the marriage is probably not going to be idyllic, to say the least.

> *Are there physical factors that may get in the way of a good marriage, aside from the general ups and downs of diabetes?*

Yes, there's male impotency, for one. There's more on this elsewhere in this book, but about a quarter of middle-aged men and some younger have an increasing decline in sexual potency.

Although it's difficult to say with any certainty, many experts do believe that this condition is probably due to neuropathy which, in turn, may be related to diabetic control as well as the length of time you've had diabetes. There may also be some sexual problems that diabetic women encounter (more fully described earlier in this chapter), despite the plethora of research (actually, non-research) that has consistently maintained diabetic women have no sexual declines in function or libido. Full understanding of all these possibilities ought to be part of every couple's premarital discussion and thinking. The questions each partner should be asking are these:

—If my husband should become impotent, am I the kind of person who can learn and be satisfied with other ways of expressing intimate feelings?

And for the man:

—If my wife has an inordinate number of sexual and urinary infections, if she has any problems at all relating to sexual expression from her diabetes, am I the kind of person who can be understanding, patient, and loving through it all?

—Can I determine the kind of person I'm marrying by the way he/ she's dealt with diabetes in the past?

In a way, you surely can. Take Bernie, who has always been totally cavalier about his diabetes, and whose blood sugar, as a result, has always careened up and down. Bernie refuses to consider the new ways of home blood sugar monitoring because he says he can "feel" when his blood sugar is high and he doesn't need any "complicated finger pricking." Bernie ignores his diabetes, in short, and already has serious complications that are directly traceable to his refusal to use judgment and care in self-treatment.

Is Bernie a dream of a good marriage risk? Well, would you marry anyone who thought it was nothing to run across busy intersections without looking for cars? Would you marry a guy who thinks Russian roulette is a super party game? Bernie is *not* every mother's dream of a good marriage risk, and it's not because of his diabetes: it's because of his denial of his diabetes.

Do people with diabetes have diabetic children?

Until very recently, the answer to this question was largely a matter of which doctor you'd spoken to. Data were scarce, controversy was rife, and two people considering marriage and a family in the face of diabetes could easily tear their hair in frustration—so wide-ranging were the guesses. As we go to press with this book, quite literally, the newest and best information comes to us from Jørn Nerup, M.D., D.Sc., Chief Physician at Steno Memorial Hospital in Gentofte, Denmark.

First of all, insulin-dependent diabetes and non-insulin-depended diabetes are inherited quite differently from each other; the hereditary element in non-insulin-dependent diabetes is much stronger than in insulin-dependent diabetes. The risk of developing insulin-dependent diabetes is only five to six percent in children who have one parent with insulin-dependent diabetes. It's not known what the risk of having a child with insulin-dependent diabetes is when two parents have the disease because there simply has not been enough research yet on the subject. Still, Dr. Nerup says he has four sets of parents who both have insulin-dependent diabetes and none of the children has diabetes.

To go further, scientists have discovered that almost a hundred percent of people with insulin-dependent diabetes also have certain gene groups which produce protein substances called HLA-DR3 and DR4 antigens (see the section on Genetic Markers for a fuller description of these gene groups). If an insulin-dependent diabetic parent is in this HLA-DR3 or DR4 group (and he/she probably is), fifty percent of the children will carry the diabetes susceptibility gene. Since only approximately five percent of those children become insulin-dependent diabetics, only about one/tenth of the carriers will *ever* develop the disease. New research is making it possible to identify high-risk and low-risk individuals in families.

To sum up and in Dr. Nerup's words: "Do insulin-dependent diabetic parents have diabetic children? The answer is rarely."

There's no absolutely sure answer. If you want to marry and have children, and diabetes is in your picture, you'll have to make your own best judgment as to the risks of producing a diabetic child—after you do some serious reading and questioning of the experts. We'll tell you this: we've interviewed, for this book, a whole lot of diabetic mothers and fathers who have produced some perfectly wonderful, diabetes-free children. Now whether those children are carriers, or will develop diabetes later in their lives, nobody yet knows. You pays your money and you takes your chances—like everybody else in life.

There's no question, the considerations are great when you're thinking marriage. Yes, diabetes can invade a marriage in an intrusive, destructive manner, but it can also have the opposite effect. Sharing the care of an illness that does not preclude living the good life can be very nurturing to a marriage. It can bind together. It can enrich. So, do not call off the wedding because one of your parents is going crazy with the irrational fear that marrying a diabetic is a sure blow to happiness. Only call it off if *you* feel that living with diabetes will be just too hard.

If you are committed to each other's care and joy, if you are knowledgeable about what's myth and what's fact in diabetes, then the chances are pretty good that you'll live a long, healthy life together. Listen—no one makes promises to any couple about to tie the knot that they'll live happily ever after; either one can be struck down by a million unexpected disasters. Diabetics who are careful and educated in the newest ways of self-care actually live a healthier life in terms of diet and exercise than most other people. Their children are taught to question the value of sugar pops and other disasters. The quality of life is somehow heightened when two people are determined not just to survive but to flower in the face of some built-in difficulties.

In the final analysis, it's up to the individuals themselves and their ability to be resilient, flexible, and loving in times of stress. The only really stupid thing any couple can do is to *ignore* the fact that one or both of them has diabetes. The illness is real. It requires adjustments and clear thinking. Given a realistic, clear-thinking couple, diabetes should not be a barrier to a good marriage.

SUGAR MOMMIES AND DADDIES: DIABETES AND PREGNANCY

Linda's Story

I think a lot about how I came through my pregnancy and I think my eventual success was due to attitude. If you think of yourself as a freak, as being abnormal and substandard as a woman and a person because you have diabetes, then that's how you'll act, and that's how other people will treat you. Diabetes isn't the only medical condition (note I don't use the word "disease": disease is what happens when you don't take care of yourself) in the world that people have. There are a lot worse things. I learned early to take care of myself. My father is a fifty-year-plus diabetic, sixty-four years old, with terrible complications because he never took care of himself (partially due to the lack of knowledge, then, on the subject). In a negative way, he's an inspiration to me to take care of myself. At ten, I started going to the Joslin Clinic Teaching Unit in Boston and then spent years as a camper and counselor at Clara Barton Camp for Diabetic Girls. Both experiences showed me I was "different" but equal and could live a normal though modified life.

I've been pregnant three times—my first, seven years ago, pre-marriage, aborted electively. My second pregnancy was planned. I knew I needed and wanted a doctor who specialized in pregnancies of women who had diabetes, and I turned to the Joslin Clinic for a reference in my area. They immediately referred me to Dr. Steven Gabbe, and when I went to see him, I was impressed with the research going on in his hospital, all the latest equipment and tests that were available. During the seven months of that pregnancy, I felt fine; with the help of a dextrometer, I kept my blood sugars within a good low range and I made weekly visits to the doctor, who gave me many tests. It was discovered that I had an extremely small amount of amniotic fluid surrounding the baby, who seemed to be growing at a normal rate.

The doctors were worried and admitted to me to the high-risk obstetrics unit of the hospital at thirty weeks, knowing they'd probably induce labor within a few weeks because they felt the baby would have a better chance of survival outside the womb. The morning I was scheduled to have a Caesarean, the baby died in utero. I'd been prepared for the worst by my doctors. The baby had "renal agenesis"—he did not have kidneys—and would not have survived anyway. I was glad mother nature took over saving both the baby and the parents a painful birth. I went through a twelve-hour induced labor and delivered a stillborn son at two in the morning. At the delivery I was given an anaesthetic and when I groggily awakened, I held my little boy for a short while. I believe, beyond all else, those few minutes helped me to understand that this one was not meant to be.

I wanted to get pregnant soon again and my doctor was supportive of those feelings. Three months later, in June of 1980, I was pregnant again, and this time I was under Dr. Gabbe's care from the beginning instead of at three months as in my second pregnancy. I was put on the insulin pump at my own request during my fourth month, and with the doctor's support, I began to feel better than ever. At thirty-four weeks I entered the hospital to be under rigid control for a month with an anticipated delivery at thirty-eight weeks. I had a Caesarean at thirty-eight weeks and delivered a beautiful, healthy 8 pound 6¾ ounce girl, Mariel Lea, with my husband present and supportive. I'd been half-expecting a Caesarean and was prepared and as self-educated as possible (through my library). It was a beautiful, happy time and we were very proud—and still are.

Things That Were difficult

—After the second pregnancy, I was so afraid that things would not work out again, though the doctors all seemed very positive that everything was okay.

—Being in the hospital for such long periods of time, away from home, husband, family, and friends, was very hard. My husband isn't one who likes hospitals, especially after the last experience, and he didn't end up visiting as much as I'd have liked.

—It was hard to be a "good diabetic" after the baby's birth because it's so difficult to find the time, with a new baby, to care for yourself.

Things That Were helpful

—I found it so reassuring to be able to talk to the doctors about the tests and to ask a million questions about everything else.

—During the second pregnancy, when there was a chance of having a premature baby, I was taken through the intensive care unit. It really helped me to see these tiny babies being so completely and wonderfully cared for, and to know that if there was a chance for this baby, it would have the best of care.

Sugar Mommies

Not too long ago, your chances of having a healthy baby would have been less than zilch. Today, they're excellent. What's that worth to a woman who has had to give up so very much because of her diabetes? Having a healthy baby is NOT something she has to give up any more.

When she first becomes pregnant, she may have more low blood sugar reactions than usual because that small round fetus is gobbling up her body's glucose. She's also probably eating less because of morning sickness, which, incidentally, her doctor can control with medication. She's advised to eat many small meals and snacks to compensate for her insulin doses. As her pregnancy progresses, her insulin needs will probably increase as the fetus grows. Adjustments must be made according to testing results.

The wisest medical heads firmly advise that you get your blood sugar in fine control quite some time *before* you even become pregnant. Those first few months of fetus growth are crucial and good development is dependent almost entirely on your good sugar control.

If you want to be a sugar mommy, be prepared to spend a whole lot of money. It's always more expensive for a diabetic woman to have a baby because there may be several hospitalizations involved, lab tests that thrive in only a money medium, and visits to the dietician, internist, eye doctor, other specialists. Your own obstetrician should be thoroughly schooled in the pregnant diabetic's special needs (more on this a little later). To find such a doctor, call your local large hospital or medical school and ask in the Department of Obstetrics and Gynecology where such an expert can be found. One new mother, speaking of costs, said her pregnancy cost her seventeen *thousand* dollars. Luckily, she had insurance to cover most of it. Is it worth it in the long run? I mean you have to work *very* hard to keep great control and you have to save up a whole lot of dollars. So, is it worth it?

—Ask Marjorie, whose Melissa just took her first step.

—Ask Karen, whose Johnny just went trick-or-treating with the older kids, gobbling down all the fun garbage that Karen was always forbidden.

—Ask Alice, whose daughter Jenny just said her first words. They were, "Oh, shit." Oh, well.

What Tests Should I Be Having During My Pregnancy?

Again, and we can't say it too often, the informed pregnant woman with diabetes must have as her doctor an obstetrician/gynecologist who treats women with diabetes *very often* if she wishes to have the proper monitoring essential in ensuring the birth of a healthy baby. Your local obstetrician may be the sweetest guy in the world, an absolutely top-notch doctor with the finest of intentions, but if he sees only one or two women a year who have diabetes he cannot be current in his education and thinking in the field. He simply does not have the patient load to merit his entire attention on pregnancy and diabetes.

Dr. Steven G. Gabbe, who is director of the J. R. Golding Division of Fetal Medicine at the Hospital of the University of Pennsylvania, is a specialist for whom I have seen coteries of women stand and applaud as he enters a room. He has shepherded well babies from women who previously have had miscarriages, malformed children, and other disasters that have come about from uninformed care of the pregnant woman with diabetes. He suggests the following testing routine to be good medical practice in dealing with a diabetic woman throughout each stage of her pregnancy. Now, these suggestions should be taken as a guide and not as gospel; your own doctor may differ somewhat in his approach. But if you are not being tested in approximately the same manner, find out why. It is entirely possible that your doctor, warm and delicious as he is, is inexperienced in the special care that you require. If this is so, find another doctor.

Ultimately, you must be responsible and informed as to your own best treatment. You must be a self-advocate and parent advocate for the baby whom you have not yet hugged. If there ever was a field in diabetes care that has grown by leaps and bounds, it is that of pregnancy and diabetes. Your success rate in producing a healthy baby should come close to approaching that of your non-diabetic sister . . . if you are a patient who is *aware.*

This is what *should* happen in terms of tests during your pre-natal care. First, all women who are pregnant and especially those women who

- are over twenty-five
- have a family history of diabetes
- have previously had a very big baby
- have had an unexplained stillbirth
- have had a baby with a malformation
- are obese
- have hypertension
- have a current yeast infection in the vagina
- have sugar in the urine

should take the simple test for gestational diabetes (diabetes that appears in women during pregnancy and may or may not go away after the child is born). If the test is to be given only once, it is best to do it late in pregnancy (between the twenty-sixth and twenty-eighth week) when the chance of developing diabetes is greater. It's a simple blood test in which the patient is given about 50 grams of sugar before having her blood sugar tested one hour later. If the sugar is normal, chances that she'll develop diabetes in pregnancy are quite small. If the sugar content is abnormal, a glucose tolerance test will probably be required to diagnose the presence or non-presence of diabetes.

If you are an insulin-dependent diabetic or if you discover during pregnancy that you have developed the disease, then your pregnancy should be accompanied by these procedures:

1. At a fetal growth of about twenty weeks, an ultra-sound test to determine fetal growth should be performed; it should be repeated about every four to six weeks to make sure the fetus is growing normally. It's painless and quite harmless, relies on high-frequency sound waves, and is usually performed in the doctor's office or in a hospital on an outpatient basis.

2. In the beginning of pregnancy, a urine culture is taken to look for urinary tract infections. This culture is taken, thereafter, every four to six weeks to be on constant guard against infections.

3. Kidney function is measured by a test called a *creatinine clearance.*

4. The amount of protein in the urine is measured at the beginning of pregnancy and measured again every month or so.

5. An eye examination is performed at the beginning of pregnancy and your doctor should check with your ophthalmologist to see how often it ought to be repeated.

6. Fetal condition is monitored, beginning at approximately twenty-eight weeks. It's a good idea to keep a chart that records the baby's activity during the day for your doctor to consider.

7. Many doctors collect *estriols,* a hormone in the urine that demonstrates the fetal health and growth. Dr. Gabbe suggests weekly measurements for a few weeks, then twice weekly for a few weeks, and, beginning at from thirty-four to thirty-six weeks, a daily measurement.

8. Amniocentesis is the test that measures, among other things, the baby's lung development. Dr. Gabbe suggests doing it at about thirty-seven and a half weeks. The test consists of inserting a fine needle into the uterus to obtain a small amount of amniotic fluid where an essence called *surfac-*

tant is found. If the surfactant is present in adequate amounts, the doctor is more confident that your baby will not develop RDS (respiratory distress syndrome). This test is often called the LS (lecithin/sphingomyelin) ratio.

9. Starting at about thirty weeks, a stress test is performed, first weekly, then twice weekly at about thirty-two weeks. The stress test's purpose is to find out if the baby will be able to withstand the rigors of labor, which involve a temporary deprivation of his/her usual amounts of oxygen and nutrients every time the uterus contracts in a "labor pain." The doctor can determine this by injecting a hormone into your body that causes you to have small contractions, similar to the real thing, and then monitoring the baby's heartbeat. Many doctors now perform "non-stress" tests that monitor the baby's heartbeat even without contractions. The purpose of the stress and non-stress tests is to help the doctor decide whether to choose a Caesarean section delivery or a rapid vaginal delivery in order to avoid stress to the baby.

10. Finally, and probably most important of all, your own self-testing for blood glucose is of paramount importance. It is this one spectacular development in the treatment of diabetes that has heralded an age of healthy babies to healthy mothers. We're talking about blood testing, not urine testing.

Understand that insulin does not cross the placenta but maternal blood sugar does, so it's critically important to keep good control during this time. The insulin you take to regulate yourself cannot directly help your baby; only your own blood sugar crosses over. If it rises, the fetus's blood sugar will also rise. If it changes dramatically, so will the fetus's sugar change. And the first two months are singularly important because many fetal organs develop during this period. That's why modern medicine asks the woman who has diabetes to try to plan her pregnancy in order to gain excellent control before she even becomes pregnant. There's a sign posted on the floor of the Mount Sinai Hospital in New York where many diabetic women come for treatment that reads: "Let Us Know If You're Even Thinking of Becoming Pregnant."

Constantly monitoring your blood ensures the almost perfect control your developing baby requires. Dr. Fredda Ginsberg-Fellner says that almost all of her patients seem to be able to gain that perfect control, even if they've never been able to do it before. Perhaps, she says, it's because there's only a limited amount of time, a set period, that one has to be meticulous. Perhaps it's because the promise of a healthy baby is such a powerful, irresistible impetus. Whatever the reason, control is possible— and essential. And control is gained through constant monitoring of blood, even if you've only gone the urine route before.

The Delivery

For many years, women with diabetes were routinely delivered by Caesarean section as much as four to six weeks prior to their due dates. Not necessarily so, anymore. With all the new testing procedures, women with diabetic pregnancies are being allowed to go closer and closer to term. In a March 1981 article in the *American Journal of Medicine,* Dr. Steven Gabbe stated that "the clinician ideally seeks a gestational age of 38 weeks with evidence of completed pulmonary maturation." Naturally, if your doctor suspects some fetal problems, he may elect to deliver your baby early. As Dr. Gabbe said: "Premature delivery is undertaken only when all signs of fetal monitoring indicate fetal jeopardy or worsening maternal hypertension or retinopathy."

The Juvenile Diabetes Foundation puts out a brochure called *Having Children ... A Guide for the Diabetic Woman* (available through your local chapter). It lists some of the guidelines that are used to decide when the baby should be delivered immediately. They are:

- a sudden, unexplained decrease in the total insulin requirements
- a marked and sustained decrease in the activity of the baby in the uterus
- a drop of 50 percent or more in the estriol determinations
- a sudden rise in blood pressure
- any significant abnormality in any of the other tests.

In the end, timing is everything. Your doctor has to decide the exact, proper moment when your baby will be ready to face the world, and then he has to bring that baby forth. Making the right decision takes informed experience.

If, of course, your diabetes is uncomplicated and there are no urgent factors present that dictate a Caesarean section, your baby can be delivered normally.

The Baby

He/she will probably be a dream.

Don't get nervous if they clap him/her in the intensive care unit for a few days. That's prudent practice and they're watching to see that nothing untoward happens. If your sugar has been elevated and passed on to the fetus, the baby's blood sugar will drop shortly after birth. It's probable that sugar supplements may be required, either orally or intravenously, and the baby must be carefully watched until it has stabilized its own blood sugar. Then again, you may have had a premature birth, and your baby will require all the sophisticated pediatric care the hospital normally provides for premature babies. It's possible that the baby may also develop jaundice, which is not difficult to treat and cure.

Now the zapper of the question: Will the baby have diabetes? Almost surely, no. Statistics are all with you—if your husband does not have diabetes and is not a carrier. Dr. Stanley Mirsky, a diabetes expert in New York who has written and lectured widely on the subject, says that the chance of your baby becoming diabetic before the age of twenty may be 1 percent and there is a less than 10 percent chance of developing diabetes sometime during his/her lifetime. Those are pretty good odds. If your husband also has diabetes, you've got a problem because the risk jumps to about a 50 percent chance of the disease developing during your child's life.

Home, James

Now you've delivered a healthy baby and have brought her home to a waiting crib, and all your troubles are over, right? Wrong. If ever a woman with diabetes needed help and support, it's now. Don't be shy. Ask for it. Demand it. If you're rich beyond all dreams of avarice, you have no problems with help. If you're not, your attitude should be, "Everyone has to chip in or I'll cry and faint a lot."

You need support—emotional and physical—until your body has a chance to recuperate from the rigors of childbirth. Try to maintain the excellent control you've been keeping, not just for the sake of the baby now, but for all of you. And don't exhaust yourself to the point of an insulin reaction. Eat your meals on time even if Junior is yelling for his. It's not terrific to pass out while alone in the house with a two-month-old; he probably won't know know what to do to help you. Many women find it helpful to leave emergency snacks in every room—including the bathroom—for quick fixes. Keep packets of sugar or cans of orange juice right on the baby's changing table so you don't have to go looking for them while juggling a full diaper.

And be prepared for your own insulin needs to drop dramatically for a few weeks soon after you've given birth. Keep in mind that you are far more active than before, with a new infant, and that should tend to cut down your insulin needs even more. Juggle, juggle, juggle—with the help of your doctor—and soon you'll be back on an even keel.

The best help of all, the very best, is your husband's love, support, and willingness to be an equal part of the parenting team (not a 25 percent part). If the last ten years of women's liberation have taught you nothing else, it should be this: fathers *need* the nurturing experience as much as mothers. What's more, they are quite capable of doing everything you can do. What's more, the baby and the father, not to mention you, will be far better adjusted and happy if Daddy learns about handling bottle supplements in the middle of the night, diapering, and cuddling.

Breast Feeding

Of course you can do it . . . if you want to. If you are healthy, apart from the diabetes, there's nothing nicer and more loving. If your baby has been separated from you for a while at birth and you have not been consistently nursing, you may have to pump your milk manually or with a breast pump to get it flowing and to keep it flowing until the baby's at your breast.

Things to watch for: If you are nursing, your insulin requirements will be less. Make adjustments accordingly. Nursing can cause sudden glucose level drops, so it's a good idea to have a carbohydrate snack, a glass of milk, or even some tea with honey before you begin to breast feed so that your blood sugar does not go blooey. Maintain your fluid intake—nursing depletes it. Maintain your diet and add about 600 to 900 calories daily because you're expending that much in milk production. Your baby will not be affected by your insulin and will not ever have insulin reactions, so stash that fear. And one last caution: Keep your breasts clean in order to forestall any chances of infection. Report irritation or redness to your doctor, who will prescribe a mild salve or antibiotic.

Some Big Questions

Does having a baby bring more medical problems to me than it does to a woman who doesn't have diabetes?

It could. Staying in good control helps a lot. Dr. Steven Gabbe says that pregnant diabetic women may have an increased incidence of pre-eclampsia (high blood pressure and urinary loss of protein). You may also develop excess amniotic fluid and more urinary tract infections. If you have retinopathy and it gets worse, often it will return to the original condition after delivery.

As long as I breast-feed, I don't need contraception—right?

Wrongo, again. Conception during nursing can happen even though it's rare. Smart money advises the diabetic woman against using birth control pills (fully explained earlier in this chapter); but even if you *have* decided to use that form of contraception, you should definitely not use the Pill while nursing.

Is there any new device that can help me to attain better control during pregnancy?

Yes, in several Boston hospitals there are studies going on which teach you to measure your basal temperature and to recognize the early signs of pregnancy. As soon as you know you're pregnant, you are fitted with a battery-operated portable insulin pump that measures out insulin subcutaneously (under the skin) much as a normal pancreas does. It's usually worn just in the critical first two months of pregnancy when many fetal organs are developing. Other doctors, including Dr. Lois Jovanovic, Assistant Professor at the Cornell Medical College, have reported benefits from the use of the insulin pump, particularly by women whose blood sugar has always fluctuated wildly.

Are certain insulins better than others during pregnancy?

Dr. Jovanovic has reported on brand-new studies advocating the use of purified insulins during pregnancy. Although insulin does not cross the placenta, antibodies to insulin do cross over to the fetus and may be a possible cause of fetal disorders. It's a good idea to start using purified insulin in early adulthood, which might lower the amounts of insulin antibodies before the childbearing years are even reached.

Are there specific diet plans for pregnant women?

Dr. Jovanovic cites an ideal diet plan (with modifications for the obese patient). In general, she says, the apportionment of calories ought to come close to 40 percent of those calories being carbohydrates, 20 percent being proteins, and 40 percent being fat. Check with your own doctor and/or nutritionist for a tailormade program for you. Adequate amounts of protein are especially important because that's responsible for tissue-building in the fetus.

Can I take my usual single shot of insulin during pregnancy?

Dr. Steven Gabbe says that split doses, usually two a day, are the normal prescription for pregnant diabetics. Some patients even take three and sometimes four shots if their individual blood sugar tests warrant these multiple doses.

Will health insurance cover the costs of home blood glucose monitoring and, perhaps, the pump, during my pregnancy?

Usually it does. The alternative to those relatively modest costs, you might point out to your company representative, could be mind-boggling hospital bills which they would have to pick up.

Can I rely on my usual urine tests during pregnancy?

No! Dr. Gabbe says that pregnant diabetics will find that their urine tests, which were usually negative, are showing considerable amounts of sugar because kidney function changes and the kidneys filter out more sugar. The pregnant woman cannot rely on urine tests now and must do an increased number of blood sugar tests to evaluate control: four or more a day, preferably.

What exactly is good control?

According to Dr. Gabbe, although it's difficult to define, fasting plasma glucose should be maintained at near 110 mg. percent and post-prandial (after a meal) at near 140–150 mg. percent. Blood sugar levels should fall no lower than 70 mg. percent. Above all, wild swings in sugar levels and frequent hypoglycemia (low blood sugar) should be avoided.

What is "gestational diabetes"?

Sometimes, there appears a special kind of diabetes in which elevated blood sugar levels occur only during pregnancy. The pregnancy intensifies a very mild diabetes, making it more obvious because the placental hormones render insulin less effective. If the disease was not a preexisting one, in however mild a form, it will probably go away once the baby is born. Naturally, gestational diabetics need the same good pre-natal care as any other kind of diabetic to ensure their baby's health. According to the *Joslin Diabetes Manual,* for half the women who develop gestational diabetes, overt diabetes can be diagnosed within fifteen years of their pregnancies.

What's the bottom line on good control during pregnancy?

According to Jane Brody of the *New York Times,* the bottom line is improved control of blood sugar. Self-testing for blood glucose can virtually *eliminate* the increased risk of fetal mishaps among diabetics. One study found that it so reduced pregnancy complications that a net saving of $5,000 per pregnancy resulted.

What's a good name for the baby?

Try "Lucky." That's what you are if you're diabetic and planning to have a baby in 1983 or thereafter. Before the new advances of home blood monitoring and pre-natal testing, you would have been better off adopting—for sure. Lucky is what you are.

And two more mothers who have diabetes—Carol and Janyce

Carol Keldea:

I not only have diabetes, I have that other dread disease, advanced maternal age. I was thirty-four when I was married, afraid to have my own baby and, I found out, too old to adopt—so they told me. I was also overweight and I had a blood sugar of 200. At thirty-eight, I decided to give it a try myself, lost 25 pounds, got my sugar down, and miracle of miracles found myself pregnant! Everyone, all my friends and relatives, told me I could lose the baby at any time.

I was told to quit work and I was terribly upset: blood sugar rocketed! The doctors and I compromised, and I worked until the thirty-second week, when it became vital to the success of the pregnancy that I enter the hospital and be monitored closely. I did what I was told, checked home blood sugar three and four times daily as well as my blood pressure. During the ultra-sound test, Jim and I saw our baby moving and what a thrill that was. The amniocentesis was rather a traumatic time, but with support from my husband and doctors, I survived it nicely.

In order to test my weekly estriol levels, I used to carry a gallon jug and a cup to work: toward the end of the pregnancy, the jug became my constant companion. Finally, October 27 arrived, the day the doctors decided would be optimum for my baby's birth because the hormone levels, lung development, and size seemed right.

My husband and I went to the labor floor, hand in hand, to await the birth of our daughter: what a joyous time to share. At 10:15 A.M., Kristin Elizabeth, 7 pounds 1 ounce and 19 inches long, was born. Crying loudly, I might add, and perfect.

Janyce Piwovar:

Now they tell you that with good blood sugar control, you can lessen the complications of diabetes. But when I was growing up (I'm thirty-two now and I've had diabetes for twenty years), the textbooks said that there was no proof that good control would lessen complications. This kind of drove me to the Eat, Drink, and Be Merry school of thought.

Well, I wasn't so merry all the time. Actually, I was manic-depressive. Most of the guys I dated only liked me when I was manic or when I was sleeping, which used to happen a lot. I'd fall asleep in my date's car, usually right after we went out to eat, because my sugar level was in outer space somewhere. I never told anyone I was diabetic because no one was to know I had an imperfection.

When I went to college, I decided to become a medical technologist because that way, at least, I could know what my blood sugars were (there were no dextrometers in 1970). I finally ended up as a pharmacist because then I could get all the needles and insulin I needed. My body was punished from my years of abuse and I always knew that if I married at all, it would have to be to a doctor, who would understand my wacky mood swings, anger, and alcoholic-like behavior.

I had many visits to the hospital for various medical problems. Whenever that happened I would always wear my white scrub coat; that way I knew I could run around the hospital to get my exercise, which no one seemed to think was important but me. What's more, with that coat, I could visit the chemistry lab to find out my blood sugars because the nurses took so long I'd have reactions. One doctor once wrote an order telling the nurse to confiscate my insulin and syringes because I was shooting up without his permission.

I never really thought I'd become pregnant: after six years of marriage to that doctor I'd finally found, I couldn't believe that I was going to be a mother. But it wasn't so simple. My obstetrician, who really knew very little about diabetes, told me to have an abortion. So did my eye doctor and my internist. I was close to being suicidal.

I changed doctors—to a wonderful specialist in diabetic pregnancies who took one look at me and said that my pregnancy would be a real cliffhanger. Was I willing to play the odds, take a chance on ending up blind *and* without a child (my eyesight, from neglect, had deteriorated badly at that point)? I was. They put me on the first primitive insulin pump, which had no safeguards and on which it was easy to overdose—I almost did.

I used to watch the Phil Donohue show, and his programs with mothers and their natural childbirths. There never was a more unnatural childbirth than mine. At thirty-three weeks, my kidneys stopped working and they performed a Caesarean section. My little son was perfectly formed externally and he had beautiful big blue eyes, but his lungs were not matured. Rushed to the intensive care nursery, he was put on oxygen, but his frail, tiny lungs collapsed, chest tubes were inserted, and he was placed on a respirator.

The nursery looked like something out of a science fiction movie and it's difficult for me even to describe the first week of Andrew's life. My postpartum depression was intensified, naturally, and I couldn't even bear to be in the same hospital room with mothers of healthy babies. My body went completely out of control and I passed out in the intensive care nursery right over my son whom I'd been anxiously watching. I couldn't sleep nights. I would sit up, watch my son breathe, and sing him old Beatles songs. A week and a half passed. My baby's lungs started to grow stronger. I'd resigned myself to his death, but it was like God saying, "You've suffered enough—Heaven can wait."

Today, Neil and I are the parents of a gorgeous, smart, and devilish little boy. Also healthy. He retains a small scar on his chest near the left armpit. My vision is quite good enough to see it, after all. The gamble paid off. I have that baby and reasonable health, which would have been better had I known enough to take care of myself from the beginning. Still, he's here, we're all here—and a happier family you can never find.

SPECIAL PROBLEMS OF WOMEN (IT ITCHES, IT HURTS, AND I DON'T LOVE TALKING ABOUT IT)

There isn't a woman alive who hasn't had at least a mild vaginal infection of some sort, and if you are a woman with diabetes, you are more prone to them. How come? The sugary urine of diabetics provides a splendid medium for vaginal yeast infections, not to mention urinary tract and kidney infections. They're generally not serious but must be tended to immediately because, as with any other infection within the diabetic system, they're harder to clear up and more potentially dangerous if they last a long time. What's crummy is that the woman with diabetes tends to blame herself for these infections, as if, somehow, her personal hygiene were somehow suspect.

Now, it's of course essential that you are aware of personal hygiene, but no one is perfect and you can't be racing to the bathroom to suds up every moment. More likely, your infection is caused by high blood sugar and not by sloppiness. Get into the habit of believing in yourself, which means to no small degree that you are as sweet-smelling, desirable, and clean as anyone else! Even if you don't put paper on strange toilet seats as your mother grimly warned you to do, you're not a slob. New evidence has it that paper on toilet seats doesn't do a thing to prevent infection, anyway.

Here, thanks to Planned Parenthood of New York, are descriptions of some common infections "down there," which often go away by themselves as suddenly as they appeared. If they don't, though, see a doctor pronto. Treatment is usually quick, non-embarrassing, and effective.

Monilia   Caused by an overgrowth of the yeast that is naturally present in the vagina, it looks like a white or cream-colored discharge—something like cottage cheese. You may also notice an odor that's similar to bread baking. It can cause itching and swelling, and in diabetes, it's almost always aggravated as the blood sugar rises. A douche that is often effective for this problem consists of a tablespoon of vinegar in a quart of warm water.

Itching Under the Breast Seems to be a common complaint of diabetic women that comes about because of a raised sugar content in the skin. Ask your doctor about a fungus powder for relief.

Other Fungus Infections Men often find them cropping up in the groin area because fungi love warm, moist places. Boxer shorts, of course, allow for more ventilation than the tight little jockey numbers and are recommended by most doctors to prevent the infections from appearing. Women ought to stick to cotton underpants that breathe and avoid tight pantyhose. Fungicides, prescribed by your doctor, are quite helpful.

Urinary Tract Infections These can often lead to more serious kidney problems, so if they're present, deal with them immediately. Such infections are often characterized by a burning sensation as you urinate, by frequent urination, by a feeling of "having to go" but then not being able to expel more than a few drops, and by pain in the lower abdomen or urinary tract itself. See your doctor right away.

Trichomonas That's the name of the organism that causes the infection. It comes with a gorgeous, foamy yellow-green discharge that doesn't have a super smell and creates itching, stinging, or genital swelling. It can easily spread to the urinary area, causing a more serious problem. It can also be passed back and forth during intercourse, so if you have "trich" and you also have a lover, he'll be clever to wear a condom during intercourse.

Crabs Yeah, yeah, it's embarrassing. They're pubic lice, usually passed by sexual contact and sometimes from infected clothing or linens. No one thinks they're cute.

Vaginal Warts Hard little bumps, often left alone by doctors if they're doing no harm. There is medication to dissolve them, or they can be removed surgically if they're large.

Herpes Infection Not so simple as the others. These are sores (like a mouth cold sore) caused by a virus, and they appear, among other places, in the genital area of both women and men. They cannot be cured, as of this writing, and they come and go; but treatment to give relief is available and all kinds of new possible cures are being worked on at this very moment.

Syphilis and Gonorrhea   Two serious genital infections usually obtained by sexual contact. Syphilis may start with a painless vaginal sore and then be followed by rashes, headaches, fever. Gonorrhea may start with a vaginal discharge, then proceed to high fever, abdominal pain, and God knows what else. Both diseases are terribly dangerous unless they're cured with penicillin or other antibiotics. And, make no mistake, both *are* curable, so get moving to do something.

As we've pointed out, you can be Ms. Clean and still develop vaginal infections because of your tendency toward sugary urine. Still, it can't help to be reasonably aware of feminine hygiene.

What's Feminine Hygiene, Anyway?

It's not a weird, romantic ritual as the television ads would have you believe. It's *not* squirting yourself up with Summer's Eve or delicious Wintergreen Vaginal Spray or any one of a number of expensive, prepared commercial products that can sometimes *cause* inflammations and severe reactions. All you have to do is:

1. Wash regularly. You don't even have to douche because the vagina cleans itself naturally. Douching more than once or twice a week definitely upsets the chemical balance of the vagina which helps ward off infection. When you bathe or shower, be sure to clean inside the outer vaginal folds where bacteria hide. Rinse carefully since soap can cause itching. Dry carefully.

2. After a bowel movement, wipe away from the vaginal opening front to back to avoid ferrying the bacteria right where it loves to grow.

3. Avoid, as much as possible, tight pantyhose, girdles, and underpants that don't breathe (like nylon ones). These don't allow enough air to circulate to keep your genital area dry, and moisture combined with a higher body temperature caused by the tight garments may aid the growth of infectious organisms.

4. See your doctor very soon if you have any signs of a urinary tract infection or a vaginal infection that doesn't get better quickly.

CAN YOU TRUST THEM AT THE HOSPITAL?

No!

Once again, it's a question of being your own best advocate. When you have a chronic disease that's so misunderstood and so replete with myths, *you probably know more than almost anyone else about your day-to-day care.* And you have to insist upon your right to exercise that care as you've learned is best for you.

Suppose, for some miserable reason, you find yourself in the hospital. You've had an accident, you need surgery, you need tests . . . something has put you there. And although the hospital should be the safest place in the world for a person whose health is in question, often it's not. There have been stories about mismanagements of diabetes in hospitals that have produced not only elevated blood sugars and insulin reactions but far more serious results, including death. Why? Naturally, no one's out to get the diabetic any more than say the bleeding ulcer patient. But absolute ignorance about diabetes, arrogant or hurried doctors, misread orders, and carelessness seem to affect the diabetic patient who needs his food on time and his insulin (or sugar source, in a reaction) absolutely *when* he needs it. And don't kid yourself that it can't happen in your hotshot, wonderful hospital center that just won an award for superiority. It can. Just listen:

—The nurse has been terrific about bringing your insulin shot on time. Only trouble is, breakfast is late because you've received the wrong tray and hospital rules say you have to wait until everyone has received her tray before yours is replaced. Bonnng! Trouble.

—You feel an insulin reaction coming on and you ask the nurse for a sweet thing *immediately* and she says, "Diabetics aren't supposed to have sweets, Mr. Smith." Bonnng! Trouble.

—The doctor visits you; knowing that you're afraid of having an insulin reaction because of the extra stress of being in the hospital, that nice person brings you sugar cubes in a little box. Ten minutes after he leaves, the dietician whisks them away, refusing to believe you, despite the fact that you're twenty-seven and reasonably sane-looking. Bonnng! Trouble.

—The doctor has left a note that the extern has permission to prescribe insulin changes if she thinks you need one. Bonnng! Trouble.

—You tell the aide you'd like some orange juice fast. She says okay and doesn't come back for half an hour. When she does, she is toting some diet ginger ale. Bonnng! You know what.

You've got to protect yourself in large institutions like hospitals. It's your responsibility. Lester Baker, M.D., chief of the Division of Endocrinology and Diabetes at Children's Hospital in Philadelphia, says that although a general practitioner in charge of a case of someone who has diabetes (on top of what she's in the hospital for) ought to confer with diabetes specialists, house staff, nurses, and nutritionists—as well as the patient herself—about her care, in a less than perfect hospital world this doesn't often happen. Here are some things you ought to do to ensure that you don't go home much sicker than you arrived, in terms of diabetes, anyway.

1. If you feel that you want to do your own blood tests (perhaps even in addition to the hospital's for your own peace of mind), mix and take your own insulin shots, or deal with any other part of your diabetes, ask for a written signed note to this effect from your doctor. Remember, he/she may not be present when you are admitted or during other parts of your hospitalization.

2. Also request written permission from your doctor to have nearby a box of Hershey bars, M & M's, orange juice cans—anything else you're in the habit of treating reactions with.

3. Make sure that you have a doctor who is familiar with diabetes (as well as the other thing you're in the hospital for) involved in your care.

4. Specifically ask the doctor how your diet or insulin should change when you have to go down for tests, when you are scheduled for surgery, etc.

5. If interns, aides, or any hospital personnel come to take your case history, and they forget to ask about diabetes, volunteer the information.

6. Check every medication you're given, every food, to make sure it's the thing that your diabetologist has agreed to.

7. Be firm if you suspect error (be nice, too; it doesn't pay to get wildly outraged). Simply refuse any further treatment until you are satisfied that your doctor's orders are being carried out.

8. Always continue to receive and take your insulin even if the dosage must be altered because of food or other changes. And if your insulin dosage has been altered prior to surgery or tests, be sure to ask the doctor to specify when your regular dosage should be reinstated.

9. Try to get your blood sugar as controlled as possible if you need surgery, *before* the surgery; but slightly high sugar is not terrible either to forestall an insulin reaction.

10. Finally, educate everyone who comes near you—especially those nurses, doctors, and other personnel who will not believe you when you say you must have food, sweets, whatever. As Dr. Baker feels, little will change until both doctors and nurses abandon the attitude that they're the only ones who know something about diabetes and the patient is simply an uninvolved object.

INSURANCE

Traditionally, people with diabetes have had a tough time getting insurance of any sort; until the mid-1940s, they were automatically rejected by virtually every insurance company. Even today, because insurance companies are in the business of making money, they are happiest to take on those customers for whom the risk of having to pay out claims is the least. But there's no question, things are easing up. The most encouraging thing about it is that there's no set policy among companies. You simply have to shop around to see which one offers the best deal for you.

You are even able to obtain, from some companies, life insurance at no higher premiums (a "standard risk" policy) if you meet certain qualifications. For instance, Leslie Spielberg, a vice president of the Underwriting Department of the Standard Security Life Insurance Company of New York (a company that has become progressively more liberal in its attitude about issuing policies to diabetics), says that if your diabetes was diagnosed after you were twenty years old; if you have no significant complications, have had the disease for fewer than fifteen years, take fewer than 100 units of insulin daily and are under competent medical care—Standard will issue a life insurance policy at no higher premium than for anyone else.

If you were diagnosed younger, or have complications, you will have to pay a premium that's higher.

In many companies, diabetics can also have health, accident, hospitalization, and disability insurance *as members of a group insurance* at no extra premiums; individual plans will undoubtedly be higher in premium and much harder to get. The group plans are better also because the employee in such a plan is not individually examined or evaluated as to health status and, once insured, the contract cannot be cancelled unless the whole group's contract is cancelled. In addition, most group plans offer major medical insurance and reimbursement, really a *must* for anyone with diabetes, who has to consider the possibility of surgery, serious illness, maternity coverage eating up a whole lot of money. A good, caring, knowledgeable insurance broker can help you to get the best for the least money.

NOW: Here comes some information we feel must be given to you in the general spirit of this book's theme, which is—be your own best self-advocate. It is little-known information, because, as you will see, most insurance companies try as best as they can to keep it from the public intelligence. Most people are not aware of their rights, don't read policies carefully (not that you'll find what follows written on any policy), and generally, cheat themselves of benefits. We caution you first! *We do not advocate* that you handle the information you're about to receive in any special way, that you equivocate or dissemble in any way when dealing with insurance companies. In short, we're not saying that lying is nice. We only say that you have a right to know your rights and then use the information in any way you choose. So here's some news you'd have a hard time finding in any other books of this nature:

In this country, there is a huge, Big Daddy computer system known as the Medical Information Bureau (MIB to those in the field). The information you provide any insurance company—or have provided in the past as to doctors or present or past illnesses automatically goes into MIB's belly and is kept for all time. Any policy you wish to buy in the future is dependent on this information. Hardly anyone knows this, as we've said, even though it's supposed to be common knowledge. Is there a legal constraint that says you really have to tell an insurance company that you have a diabetes condition (or a heart or cancer or sickle cell anemia condition)? There is not. New York State law, and it's the same in most other states, protects you; the only way insurance companies and the Medical Information Bureau can find out about your health is if you tell them.

Now naturally, if you just leave blank the part on the form that specifically asks you about "sugar in the urine" or diabetes or whatever, you're not going to get the policy. But suppose, for a moment, you exercise your right to withhold the information that you are a diagnosed diabetic. You buy life insurance and *within two years* you die from the condition (highly unlikely; we're just giving you a "for instance"). The insurance company has the right, and will surely perform an investigation, to determine if you had the condition before you took the policy. If they discover that you did, they can refuse to pay up on the policy, and instead would refund to your estate the total of all premiums paid plus interest.

But suppose you died *after* you'd had the policy for two years. In most states, your heirs to the insurance are safe; the insurance company must pay up, *even if you have misrepresented your state of health.* The two years, by the way, is known as the "contestability period" and may differ from state to state.

Suppose you have health insurance and you get sick as a result of the diabetes you have not told anyone about, and you wait until after that two-year period to make a claim. You have to collect. What's more, whether the company has paid, or refused to pay because they've found out within the contestability period that you did indeed have a preexisting condition, they may not notify the Medical Information Bureau on the disposition of these claims.

The Bottom Line: There is no law that insists you have to tell an insurance company about any illness or condition you may have. If you have never told any other company before when you've applied for a policy, the Medical Insurance Bureau has no record on you—and neither will your new company.

Again, please understand: we're not telling you to be less than honest; we're simply quite interested in your knowing every right and advantage that's at your disposal.

A CONTROVERSIAL LOOK AT JOB HUNTING—DO THEY HAVE TO HIRE ME?

Almost always, the answer is Yes. But you've all heard the stories.

Item

Liz never lied in her life. When she applied for a job as a receptionist in a lawyer's office, she answered Yes to the question, "Have you any physical disabilities?" She didn't get the job . . . even after she explained that her diabetes was fully controlled and she was probably healthier than anyone else in the office. "We can't take a chance on startling our clients if you should feel suddenly ill," was the response.

Item

Buddy was going to dental school. During the summer, he applied for a job with the sanitation department to make some badly needed tuition money. He told them about his diabetes. The answer was No. "It makes the other men nervous," they said. It seemed collecting garbage was out for a diabetic.

Item

Lynne called a state-run agency for a job, mentioned her diabetes when asked about medical history, and was told she was a "handicapped person" and could be hired under that label. She hated it. The label, the idea. She told them to shove the job.

Okay, here's the scoop. If you're qualified to be a brain surgeon, cab driver, or ice-cream maker—go to it and try to get the job. There are very few opportunities that are not available to you and which the law denies because you are a diabetic. The ones that are out?

—The Federal Aviation Administration denies airline pilot licenses to insulin-dependent diabetics.

—The federal government prohibits diabetics from entering the armed services, driving trucks or buses in interstate commerce.

—Sometimes, state and local governments prohibit diabetics from entering police-type work.

Before we begin on the controversial stuff, there are a few points to make.

—It really makes sense, even if you're not forbidden by law, to avoid any job that you may reasonably expect to get either you or someone else into trouble should you have a reaction. This might include fixing telephone poles, leading scuba-diving expeditions, or being a firefighter. It does *not* make sense to exclude jobs that fearful physicians, parents, friends advise you against because there's a chance in a million that you may have an insulin reaction and cause an accident. No one has the right to "protect" you against living the fullest and most creative life *you yourself reasonably feel* you can handle. Of course, be aware of your limitations; but never be caught between well-meaning yet often misguided caution and your own self-confidence.

—You may be a victim of job discrimination no matter what the written law says. Very few people fight City Hall and prospective employers seem to count on it. Therefore, smart money says that you ought to protect yourself in any legal way possible—even if it doesn't sound too nice. Which brings us to the part you won't read in any other book because it's not the traditional, safe advice that's easy to give.

Most articles you'll read on the subject, certainly every book on diabetes we ever read, tell you to be up front, straight on, Honest George—every euphemism in the dictionary that means be fearlessly candid in job interviews. We disagree. It's surely honorable and admirable to lay all your cards on the job interview table; but judging from conversations we've had with many, many job hunters, it's not the most self-serving thing to do. And like it or not, self-serving is what you have to be sometimes, especially with people who are prejudiced, ignorant, or simply unwilling to take a chance on anything at all that smacks of "different."

There is absolutely no question about it: you have a better chance of getting a job if you do not announce your diabetes than if you do. What's more, there is absolutely no legal compulsion that requires you to disclose the fact of your diabetes unless you want to be part of a company's affirmative action program for recruiting and promoting "handicapped" workers. We're not telling you to lie. We're simply saying that you do not have to give ammunition to people who know nothing about the uniqueness of you, the nature of diabetes, or your motives. And personnel departments of organizations are not known to be particularly insightful or understanding. They just don't want to make waves, for the most part. So, given an applicant who's mediocre and undiabetic versus an applicant who looks as if he might shine and who has diabetes, they'll go for the mediocre every time.

After you've been hired and have proved your worth, it's a good idea to begin to share the fact of your diabetes quietly with your co-workers, even your boss. Once the real you, the person is valued, the illness becomes quite secondary. And it's always better not to have to keep a secret. Also, of course, it's wonderful to know that people around you know what to do, should you have an insulin reaction.

Douglas Pavgner is a member of the New York Association of Insulin-Dependent Diabetics (AIDD). He was looking for a job in journalism but met with a "Don't call us, we'll call you" every time he talked about diabetes. So he stopped talking diabetes and started talking journalism—exclusively. He got the job. After he was hired, he told his boss he had to eat on time because he was diabetic. Eating on time when deadlines are looming is a rarity in a press room and most of his fellow workers had become resigned to missed dinner hours. Enter Douglas: the editor-in-chief has been impressed with this fledgling reporter who now tells him that eating on time is a personal requirement. "Sure, no problem," says the editor. So now Douglas—and a whole lot of happier co-workers also—are assured a dinner hour.

If Doug had mentioned, even alluded to the importance of mealtimes before he's had the chance to show his worth, he'd just never have gotten that job. Simple as that. So you fight fire with fire. Wherever there are people who are quicker to say No than Yes because they are fearful of what they don't understand, it is in your best interest to protect yourself. And that's the way the world goes, pretty-sounding or not.

Funny—once you're part of a group, an organization, a workplace, most co-workers seem delighted to help, to do what they can if you need them. Lin Campbell, another member of AIDD, says she's told everybody with whom she works: "Look, I probably won't have any problems, but there may come a time when I need a quick sugar lift and I don't feel strong enough to get a Coke so I may need you to help me. Please don't think anything of it. I'll share the Coke with you, honest. And," continues Lin, "turns out that my assistant reads me better than I can myself. She'll say, 'Hmmm, your eyes look a little glazed, you slurred that last word—would you please test your blood?'"

What if you've been above board and are denied a job and you're sure it's because of your diabetes. Have you any recourse? You bet you do:

1. Title V of the Federal Rehabilitation Act passed in 1973 by Congress says that the executive branch of government, businesses with federal contracts or subcontracts of more than $2500, and all programs and activities that receive federal subsidies must not discriminate against the handicapped. That takes care of major business involved with the government.

2. There are also state anti-discrimination laws that protect your right to work in all state businesses—not just those funded by the state—but the laws are different in each state. Want to know about your state's laws? A book entitled *The Law and Disabled People: Selected Federal and State Laws* can be obtained for $6.50 from the Supt. of Documents, U.S. Government Printing Office, Washington, DC 20402 (ask for stock no. 040-000-00432-7). It lists these state laws and tells which agencies enforce the laws if you need help.

3. Talk to an Equal Employment Opportunity Commission (EEOC) person (Tel.: 202-756-6040), who will try to resolve your problem informally first, and then very formally as she/he tells you how to file a complaint with the EEOC.

4. Talk to your union, if you belong to one, or any employment group: Perhaps they may have some ideas—and even a lawyer to champion your cause.

5. Talk to people at the local Juvenile Diabetes Foundation, who will probably be able to point you in the right direction for help and advice.

6. Finally, if all else fails, you're absolutely intent upon not being taken advantage of, and you have some dollars to spend on the effort, hire your own lawyer. He/she has greater clout than you do in convincing an employer it would be to his benefit to get rid of his evil, discriminatory practices. As a matter of fact, even if you don't have big bucks, you're still entitled to a legal aid lawyer provided by the state free of charge.

However you handle it, know that you have a right not to be discriminated against because of your diabetes. That doesn't mean you have to get a job where there are other applicants as qualified as you who perhaps are able to convince the boss of their superior characteristics—just *because* you have diabetes. It's a competitive world and you may lose out because you're not as good, convincing, or blond as the other applicants. But if you have a visceral feeling that it's your diabetes that was the stumbling block, be militant, be less than candid next time around, be your own self-advocate . . . as we've been saying all along in this book.

Don't Cry Wolf

The best thing you can do for yourself as a young working person is to stay healthy so you do not have to miss any more work than is absolutely necessary. If you want to have people think that a person with diabetes is as capable and responsible as any other working person, you'll bend over backward not to miss any more time from work *than is absolutely necessary.* Not only are employers more understanding about days off when you have a wonderful attendance record, but you have to think of yourself as a person who represents a population. If you're considered a goof-off or a "sick" diabetic, you color the atmosphere for everyone with diabetes who comes after you.

The Ten Commandments of the Insulin-Dependent Diabetic— And Don't You Forget Them

1. Thou shalt honor thy Diabetes. Well, maybe not honor it. *Pay attention* to it is more like it.

2. Thou shalt not Transgress against thy Diet, thy Exercise, or thy Insulin Shots.

3. Thou shalt not covet thy Neighbor's Blood Sugar. Okay, thou can covet it. But don't let it get thee crazy.

4. Thou shalt not bear false witness to thy doctor; if thou smoked the Marijuana and ate the Nesselrode pie, admit it, so thy doctor doesn't prescribe wrongly.

5. Thou shalt not pay homage to false gods like Urine Sugar Tests, which can be notoriously fickle; honor, instead, the Home Blood Glucose Test.

6. Thou shalt not steal, rape, or murder. It will probably only give thee an Insulin Reaction, anyway.

7. Thou shalt not kill thyself with gastronomic or Olympian iniquities.

8. Thou shalt not commit too many secret infringements or thy Hemoglobin A1c Test shall find thee out.

9. Thou shalt not be a pain in the ass about thy Disease, using it for a ready excuse to miss thy Labor, thy Appointments, or thy Good Times.

10. Thou shalt be a Self-Advocate, heeding the words of thine own education and conscience above all other words.

TIPS AND TOUTS FOR ADULTS

From Carl Burns:

I find purchased lancets crude and painful; I feel that the Monojet Autolet lancets make large holes and yield far more blood than necessary. Solution? Make your own! A nearly painless, precision lancet can easily be made from a used Monojet half-cc. syringe. Here's how:

Cut off the end of the yellow protective cap. Replace the cap on the syringe body. The fine needle will protrude through the cut-off end of the cap and the cap will limit the depth of penetration of the finder prick. File, sandpaper, or cut off more or less of the cap to obtain the exact depth of penetration needed. A generous drop of blood can easily be obtained by holding the syringe barrel as one holds a pencil, positioning the needlepoint against any opposite hand fingerpad, and rolling the two hands together without thinking about what is happening. The prick wound will heal promptly and there is no after-pain as with the Autolet. Exchange the syringe needle and barrel for a "new" used one, weekly.

From a British doctor:

Fingers need be no more than "socially clean" when extracting blood. One thing to avoid is the residue of any fruit juice or other simple saccharide on the hands. I never sterilize or use alcohol on my homemade lancets or even on my finger, and I'm testing up to ten times daily. What works for me may not work for others. I am not recommending any of the above for anyone, only describing what I do for myself, alone. (NOTE: That's all we can ask. But you'd be surprised how much it helps others to hear what you've devised that works for you—that's the real reason for this book.)

From Arlene Borish:

My son keeps small cans of soda and juice in his car for emergencies. During the snowy weather, I pack an emergency bag for him of nuts, raisins, peanut butter, crackers, regular soda, candy—anything that won't spoil—for his car. I worry silently and pray a lot.

From Sandra Hower:

When I'm going on a trip, I always call ahead to the hotel or the motel to see if they can make provision to keep my insulin cool. That way, I don't have to worry about it spoiling while I'm having fun in the sun.

From Dr. Robert Selig:

Find out from your doctor what you should be paying for an item: for instance, a patient of mine told me that she paid $45 for an Autolet and you can get them for $22. Another patient told me that her druggist charged her more money for the two-drop Clinitest than she paid for the one-drop Clinitest. Now the pill's identical in both—only the chart differs, and the price should not be different. I told her to buy the one-drop version and I'd give her a chart.

The low-dose insulin gauges with a 27½ gauge needle are the thinnest and least painful for your shots. They have a coating that makes them slide in easily, also. Ask for the low-dose microfine needles put out by B-D (Becton, Dickinson), and have your doctor use them on your kids for immunization, allergy shots—everything. (Remember that the higher number needles are thinner than the lower; 27½ gauge is thinner than 22.)

And here's a trick to make the Autolet less painful. It's wonderful, gives a perfect jab every time, but when it's very sharp, it penetrates perhaps more deeply than it has to. Hold it a little loosely, not right up to the fingertips but a bit farther away—just so it jabs you a little. It does not have to be held up directly to the fingertip.

From Linda Last:

The disease carries with it a great sense of frustration, anger, aloneness, and powerlessness. The answer at these times is human contact. When I get these "diabetic fears and obsessions," I need to talk, and I find that the more I let people know about my condition and its side effects, the more easy they and I feel with myself. It also makes me far less angry with them when they ask questions about diabetes.

From Barbara Guille:

I say No when I fill out a job application and it asks if I have any diseases. I know I'll never get the chance to prove myself if I say Yes. After I'm safely placed, everybody ends up knowing and not caring.

From Sandy Kupersmith:

You *can* bargain down the price of supplies for diabetics. If you buy anything in bulk, they'll usually knock the price down, and you need the stuff anyway.

The directions in the Autolet say you have to change the little yellow platform at the bottom of the device with each shot. That's baloney! If you ask anyone who manufactures it they'll tell you that, theoretically, when a doctor uses it with a lot of different people, it ought to be changed more frequently. However, alcohol is quite cleansing, and I have patients who have never changed the platform.

From Clara Ducham:

Don't refrigerate the vial of insulin you're currently using. When you use insulin that is cold, the body takes longer to absorb it, which is why you may see lumps at the injection site.

Take extra care during periods of high temperature and humidity.

You may have to eat more and/or take less insulin because of the strain the weather creates for your body.

From Lynda Kucko:

I find religion a great help for me—particularly the scriptures. One that seems to relate directly to my problems with my diabetes has *always* lifted me up. This is it, or part of it, anyway: II Corinthians, 12:8–10

> My grace is sufficient for you, for my power is made perfect in weakness. Therefore I will boast all the more gladly about my weaknesses, so that Christ's power may rest on me. That is why, for Christ's sake, I delight in weaknesses, in insults, in hardships, in persecutions, in difficulties. For when I am weak, I am strong.

From Lenora Stanton:

I put a *big* sign on my bulletin board with the ambulance number and my husband's number and my mother's number on it. My small children can dial a phone and they know exactly what to do if they can't wake me up.

Blue Cross and Blue Shield covers the cost of an insulin pump if a doctor prescribes it.

From Sharon Dukess:

When I go to a restaurant with my husband who is diabetic, he hates to call attention to himself by asking the waiter to bring something back that has appeared on his plate and which he cannot eat. I always take the rap for him, saying: "Could you please change this coleslaw with sugar for some plain salad because my diabetes says I can't eat sugar." I think, eventually, he'll come to see that waiters don't look cross-eyed at people who have special dietary needs and, someday, he'll do it for himself.

From Sally Risenbaum:

I got ready for my baby six months before I got pregnant. I exercised, got my glucose in control, ate only those things that were terrific. My doctor says he's certain that it helped in producing the super-kid we now have.

If you are having anxiety—see a shrink! Never, never feel dumb or self-conscious about getting psychological help for psychological problems. If your foot hurts, you see an orthopedist, don't you? It's *common* and quite normal for diabetics to worry excessively about blindness, impotence, deformity, and death. A psychiatrist or other skilled analyst can help you, as she did me, to get to the bottom of my fears, which were crowding in my life. I can't think of any tip that is more valuable for a diabetic: it saved my life, I think. Stress can kill, especially when you have high blood sugar.

From Karen Quinn:

Check with your doctor, but recently I had surgery and my doctor says I came through so well because proper attention was paid to my insulin requirements during this critical time. He ordered that I have *half* the usual amount of insulin on the morning of the surgery and an intravenous solution of glucose. After the surgery, my blood sugar was closely monitored to see when and what additional amounts I needed.

From Margorie Katz:

Always check the ingredients list on any product in the supermarket. When I'm shopping for my husband who is diabetic, I shop with a small calculator to quickly figure calories or percentages of ingredients. For instance: something that says it has only 10 calories an ounce sounds pretty reasonable. But when you're figuring a 12 ounce bottle, you're talking about 120 calories, which equals three fruit exchanges or almost eight teaspoons of sugar.

From Jon Cassavetes:

Every time I throw out a pair of sneakers that are too used to wear any more, I feel that I've done something for my disease. There's no question in my mind that exercise makes me eat better, take better care of myself, and feel better, as well as lowering my insulin needs. Start out slowly, listen to your body, and develop your body. You're more than a pancreas—you've got legs and arms and a heart also! Someone once wrote a book about diabetes called *Borrowing Time.* I couldn't disagree more. I'm on my own time, not borrowed time, and exercise allows me to use that time to the fullest.

SUGAR SPOUSES

How is it to be married to someone with diabetes? Does anyone else in this whole world understand your problems and your victories? The only way to find out was to share stories. One day, over coffee and fruit, a bunch of us got together and talked non-stop. It was a cathartic, nourishing experience that none of us will ever forget.

How is it to be married to someone with diabetes? This is how it is.

Lucy Bergen's husband is getting her *very* nervous. He's been going to the same doctor, a general practitioner, for over twenty years. The doctor takes a blood sugar reading every six weeks and doesn't seem at all concerned that Mr. Bergen's blood sugar has wild fluctuations between 86 and the high 300s. Home blood glucose monitoring? Not necessary, says the trusted old doctor. Lucy wants her husband to see a diabetes specialist, but Gil loves his doctor and is comfortable with him. Also, he hates the idea of testing his own blood. Lucy, as I said, is very nervous . . .

Sandi Saranoff's husband gets her angry as well as nervous. Bob's just had a kidney transplant and it wasn't easy to make the decision to do it, or live through the trauma of the operation. Now it's over, Bob seems fine but still won't tell anyone at work about his diabetes. He feels it could injure his career. So Sandi has to be the one who makes up the lies when a friend or fellow worker calls Bob and he can't talk because he's having a mild reaction. "Uh, he has this stomach virus, he can't come to the phone," she'll say. She loves Bob and would do anything for him, but frankly she resents having to tell lies. And also, she's terrified that he'll have a reaction at work and no one will know what to do . . .

Ginger Evans works with her husband. She's a nurse and Donald's a doctor, and they're a perfect team except for the fact that Ginger feels she has to watch Donald too carefully. Sometimes he gets so wrapped up in his work and his patients that he doesn't follow his own advice and, as a result, his diabetes is not under the control it should be. He doesn't eat on time and sometimes he even forgets to take his insulin shot on time. "There have been days when I have to tell him who he is, who I am, and where he is," says Ginger. "I mean—I *shouldn't* have to do that." . . .

Marci Ryder has diabetes and Ben Ryder is the most supportive husband in the world. He says the extra expense of being married to a diabetic just has to be cranked into the budget like the telephone bill and the food bill, "but there have been lean times when we've ridden along with just one package of syringes left and worried about where the money was going to come from for the next package." Marci's on the pump and Ben says that it's made a big difference in her moods, which seemed to fluctuate an awful lot as her blood sugar levels went up and down. "Some husbands complain that their wives have premenstrual syndrome," chuckles Bill. "Well, I have it both ways—premenstrual syndrome *and* diabetic grumpiness." . . .

It's not always easy to be married to someone who has insulin-onset diabetes. There are the tensions that every marriage has plus the peaks and the valleys of diabetes that both share. Because, make no mistake, if one person has the disease, both people have the side effects.

"It's funny," says Lucy. "You tend to blame the damn thing for everything. My child was born with a cleft lip. We never really talked about it in terms of Gil's disease but I know it's on his mind. Actually we did talk about it once. Very casually. I know Gil has it on his mind. And the first time I held the baby, I found myself crooning, 'Oh, I'm sorry ... I'm so sorry.' Now diabetes probably had nothing at all to do with the baby's birth defect, but both of us, secretly, think about it from time to time."

In the beginning it's golden days, as in the best of marriages. You're both young and strong and can beat the world, and surely diabetes, to its knees. Big deal—diabetes. We'll just take it as it comes—you take your shots and I'll live my life as I always have. Right? Well, right, until the first reaction.

"He sounded like Moon Man on the telephone when I happened to call home," says Sandi. "I didn't know what was up and I raced back from work. I thought I'd left a husband home with a little cold—and here was a *zombie* on the phone! I'd never seen a reaction but, boy, I knew it when I saw it. The bedroom was covered with glasses of orange juice and Coke which I tried to pour down him, by the time it was all over. So don't tell me, anyone, that diabetes is not a problem in marriage. Maybe it's not a problem but it certainly is a factor. When I find my husband almost incoherent, and I have to deal with it, it has to be a factor."

Some families tell you it's a breeze. Some say it's a chore. You're constantly watching for signs, say the sugar spouses. You can have the best marriage in the world, but if your husband's hand has pins and needles one day, you're both sure it's the beginning of neuropathy—even though *your* hand is always falling asleep on you. And sugar spouses read the marriage manuals like other modern young marrieds and they *know* that it's not really so unusual if a man is impotent occasionally. After all, stress does funny things to you and he's been working so hard on that new account and all ... still, still, could it be the beginning of the *real* impotence that some diabetic men have? And, what's more, could the fact that he couldn't achieve erection be due to his terror that he one day will, might, have penile neuropathy? I mean, how do you know what's real and what comes from tension and anticipation?

"I'll tell you something I firmly believe," says Sandi. "I think that once a diabetic and his spouse get through five to six years of marriage, they're absolutely committed to each other. Their marriage is stronger than *anyone's.* Are you kidding? You stick with the problems for so long, you learn how to really love. And your relationship is different from your friends' relationships. For instance, the things most people fight about, money, helping each other around the house—we don't. There are other things more important than if we can see a show this week.

"I think you get to appreciate true, good values more if you live with a diabetic spouse. I met Bob when I was sixteen. My mother said, 'What are you getting into?' My friends told me I was nuts. But I didn't listen and I'm glad. Of course, when we go on an automobile trip, I feel like taking the whole fridge along—just in case we get stuck on the road. And I worry about him dying young and leaving me alone. That's scary. He doesn't express his fears to me because he doesn't want to upset me. All in all, with all the problems, I think we're stronger together than any marriage that deals with superficialities. We deal with heavier stuff. And, believe me, we make every day count because of it."

Sometimes, it's the person with the diabetes who has problems with marriage—aside from the diabetes. Gil Bergen feels guilt because he can't buy his wife a new coat and if he didn't have to spend money on his diabetes equipment, he could. So he goes without his Tes-Tapes for a week and Lucy becomes furious. "Are you *crazy*?" she exploded one day, when she realized how he was economizing. "Do you think I want a new coat more than I want you to test your blood sugar?"

Thirty insulin pump catheters cost $60 and they last two months, so Marci Ryder tries to economize on her choices of meats for the family—and she feels guilty that three months have gone by and steak hasn't graced the Ryder table.

"Who the hell cares about steak?" says Ben. "If I wanted steak, I'd have married an heiress."

Still, there are the quiet moments in the night when Marci dreams sirloin. And it's then that she hates her diabetes the most, when she thinks it's depriving her family of the little extras in life.

Some spouses of diabetics have the hardest time with friends. Sandi and Bob were invited to dinner by someone they'd met in the hospital when Bob had his kidney transplant. All went well until dessert. The hostess served sherbet. Pink sherbet. Really luscious-looking, cool and pepperminty-looking sherbet. Irresistible.

"I couldn't stand it," says Sandi. "Bob took some and I didn't want to emasculate him by telling him not to even though I knew his blood sugar would go over the wall in an hour. The next day, I couldn't resist asking her what she was thinking as she served sherbet to a person who'd just had a kidney transplant for diabetes complications.

" 'Well, it wasn't ice cream,' she answered. 'I thought the problem was in eating ice cream.' "

"You don't want to be a mother to your husband," muses Sandi. "And you don't want to be a shrewish nag, either. But sometimes he does something that will really hurt him and even though you know it's *his* disease, and he has to be responsible for it, you just can't divorce yourself from the situation because you love him more than your life. So you try to keep your mouth shut when you're invited out to dinner and dinner is late . . . *one hour late.* Now, one hour's not so much to anyone else but I could kill the hostess for that one hour. She *knows* Bob has to eat on time. She's just forgotten. I think it's unforgivable. And then, I think, God—what the hell—it's not so unforgivable. She's busy with her party, she can't be thinking all the time of diabetes. So this is what I do: *I* get up (because Bob won't do it, he's so afraid of being rude), and I say, 'Listen, I haven't had a bite since morning. Would you mind if I just go to your fridge and get a piece of fruit till dinner is ready?' Then I get two pieces of fruit, and casually drop one on Bob's lap."

The fruit trick is one that Ginger Evans knows well. She also knows the long-distance call trick.

"When Donald is particularly overbooked and he doesn't have a minute for himself—not even to take his snack—I'll go into the examining room when he has a patient and say, 'Doctor, you have a long-distance call.' He'll excuse himself from his patient, and I walk with him into the side room where we keep snacks and juice and stuff, and I *make* him sit down for the snack he's not had time for. Yes, it bothers me that sometimes I have to act so bossy, but he's the most important person in the world to me and I can't ignore his needs—even when he does. Look, he makes it up in kind, don't worry.

"I think a man who has diabetes has to be the kindest, most loving, most fine husband in the world. He has had the experience of feeling very ill—and of having you stand by him. He knows what commitment means when he sees it in you. He only *wants* to do for you when you feel sick, when you need him. It's a mutual thing—it's not gratitude. I would marry him again, and again, and again—even knowing what I know about this lousy disease. I think diabetes binds two people together. Look, sometimes I get wild-crazy that he's obsessed with his blood sugar, his pancreas. It's just not natural to be preoccupied with your pancreas. But then, we laugh about it, and go on. It can be done. I know I sound like a soap opera when I say: 'I married a diabetic and survived.' But I did. And I will."

So there it is. Although the divorce rate is high among diabetics, it's also high among non-diabetics, so healthy pancreases promise nothing. Sugar spouses learn to live lovingly and peacefully with the "something that just doesn't go away," as one diabetic's spouse phrased it. And if high blood sugar is always an issue, there are also all the other human issues that make two people fall in love. That's the cement, that's the reason for marriage. You have to be strong and of a certain philosophical bent to bind yourself to someone who has a chronic disease. But the disease is not the dimple, or the blueness of eye, or the quickness of wit that made you love your sugar spouse.

5 COMPLICATIONS, TREATMENTS, NEWEST RESEARCH

THE WORST THAT CAN HAPPEN ...

OKAY, Let's have it. What's the worst that can happen? What are the complications of diabetes?

Every diabetic knows that bad things happen to very good, very careful people, and even with meticulous control complications of diabetes can occur. However, it is certainly true that more and more research seems to indicate severe complications are most often linked up with poor control rather than with good control. If you are a juvenile diabetic, one who presumably has gotten the disease fairly early in life, you have a better chance of forestalling and maybe even eliminating these complications if you *consistently* maintain as near a normal blood sugar count as possible. The sooner you start doing this, reporting symptoms to your doctor whenever you observe them, educating yourself about the problems that may occur, the better all-around chance you have.

Researchers all over the world (a medical SWAT company, if you will) are working daily on new ways to help insulin-dependent diabetics not only to live more comfortably but to live more hopefully that someday soon the disease can be stopped dead in its tracks—as polio and smallpox have already been stopped. This chapter, then, will tell you about some of the more prevalent complications of diabetes; what you can do to avoid and/or deal with them; and finally, what's down the road in scientific research toward balms, preventatives, and cures.

Eyes

Ask any diabetic: the complication that's most feared is blindness. And with good reason. Diabetes is one of the main causes of partial visual loss and blindness in the United States. Dr. Francis L'Esperance, Jr., Associate Professor of Clinical Ophthalmology at the College of Physicians and Surgeons, Columbia University, says that the grim statistics before the most recent advances in eye care show that 28 percent of all diabetics between the ages of thirty and fifty will become blind and that 86 percent of diabetics with retinopathy will become blind. However, with the advent of treatment so new that no recent statistics reflecting their success have yet been compiled, Dr. L'Esperance suggests that the picture is much brighter. That's encouraging but hardly comforting. The fact remains that diabetics who have had the disease for five years or longer are still far more likely to develop visual disorders and even blindness than those people who do not have diabetes.What can go wrong?

Diabetes can damage sight in several ways, but usually it affects the area of the eye known as the retina. When the small blood vessels of the eye that nourish the retina deteriorate, they can no longer supply all the oxygen and nutrients the retina requires for its good health. When this happens first, and the condition is relatively mild, it's known as *background retinopathy.* Tiny bulges in the walls of the retina's blood vessels appear (these are microaneurysms) and fluid begins to "ooze," says Dr. L'Esperance. Often treatment is not needed except when the fluid collects in the central part of the retina, called the macula, where it might cause a blurring of vision.

In many cases the retinopathy goes no further and affects only the blood vessels contained within the retina. Many people, indeed, have no symptoms at all, and that's why it's essential to have regular visits to the ophthalmologist. Dr. Arnall Patz, professor and chairman of the Department of Ophthalmology at the Wilmer Institute, Johns Hopkins University School of Medicine and Hospital, says that unfelt changes in the eye may be the first sign that there's something wrong with a patient who isn't even aware of having diabetes. "I have seen patients who, on their first visit, had retinopathy that prompted the blood sugar studies that first revealed their diabetes mellitus."

If diabetic retinopathy gets worse, it progresses to the next stage, which is called *proliferative retinopathy.* Here, abnormal new blood vessels form in and around the retina (neovascularization), bringing with them potentially disastrous threats to sight. These new vessels are delicate and can hemorrhage, bursting and bleeding into the vitreous humor, the clear gel that fills the center of the eye. This blocks or scatters the light to the eye, making the patient sightless. Scar tissue can form, which also reduces vision much like a lightshade that has been pulled down to block the light. And sometimes, scar tissue can contract and pull on the retina, which detaches it and also causes partial or total blindness. A pretty dim picture, in every sense of the word.

But if there are serious eye problems connected with diabetes, there is also marvelous, tangible progress that has been made in their treatment.

One of the new techniques brightening the picture for diabetics is known as *photocoagulation,* says Dr. Patz; this is a process that converts light rays to heat, which produces a thermal burn (a coagulation). A laser is aimed at oozing blood vessels: the concentrated light destroys the abnormal capillaries and seals them off (usually a painless procedure).

Sometimes the laser is used in scatter therapy, by which retinal mass is reduced to what its normal blood supply can handle. Here, "you're literally burning up less critical areas of the retina to spare the more vital, ventral area," says Dr. Patz. "The patient will have from five hundred to two thousand individual coagulations, scattered like polka dots around the retina." And even though the laser scattering technique, which makes many small burns pan-retinally, does not hit the vessels directly, it causes those vessels to close and stop bleeding—and the retinopathy to clear.

But photocoagulation is not a cure, Dr. Patz cautions. Although a comprehensive fifteen-hospital study known as the Diabetic Retinopathy Study showed that half to a third of patients with moderate or severe retinopathy were helped by photocoagulation, some patients were not treatable. Moreover, although the new process greatly reduced the risk of serious complications it did not eliminate the risk entirely. Therefore a large ongoing area of research is concerned with finding out methods to prevent abnormal blood vessel growth completely, as the best means of controlling retinopathy.

There is another recent advance in treatment of eye problems, which is known as *vitrectomy.* Since you can only use photocoagulation up to a point, if there is still massive bleeding that doesn't clear up by itself, the ophthalmologist can insert a small tube into the eye to suction out the bloody vitreous fluid and replace it with sterile, saline fluids that transmit light. Eventually, the body will replace this fluid with its own clear fluids. The success rate, depending on the extent of the hemorrhaging is improvement in about 50 to 60 percent of the cases.

One of the eye complications of diabetes is a form of glaucoma that can come when a patient is still very young, if he's had the disease for a number of years and particularly if he's had poor glucose control. A brand-new treatment for this glaucoma, which was previously untreatable and resulted in blindness, has been developed by Dr. L'Esperance. It involves a blue-green, carbon dioxide laser beam that can drill a microscopic hole into the eye in order to drain off accumulated fluid. Because the new laser can vaporize tissues without causing hemorrhages, says Dr. L'Esperance, and can cauterize blood vessels as it goes along, this eye problem, up till now hopeless, can today in most cases be managed.

Is there anything that the patient can do for him/herself to avoid eye problems? Absolutely. Although even following all the rules is no guarantee of avoiding complications, as we've repeatedly said throughout this book, it surely increases your chances of success. And those rules are:

—*Stop Smoking:* Dr. L'Esperance suggests that the vasoconstrictive nature of tobacco cause the peripheral blood vessels in the eye to contract under stress. This is not helpful for blood vessels that are already more fragile from the diabetes itself.

—*Keep Your Blood Pressure Within Acceptable Limits:* "Like acid eating away at your car's battery, hypertension or high blood pressure can actually blow out fragile blood vessels," says Dr. L'Esperance. "Internists are learning that when they see a patient with high blood sugar and retinopathy, the first thing they should do is try to lower that pressure to a point where the patient will not have adverse effects. Sometimes, lowering a high blood pressure fifty points or more makes retinopathy almost 75 percent better."

Keep Your Blood Sugar Within Normal Ranges: Almost all eye specialists agree that sugar levels are closely associated with eye problems. Although it's not always possible to do, no matter how you try, it's highly preferable to keep blood sugar within normal ranges (below 140 mgs. fasting, and below 200 mgs. after eating).

See Your Ophthalmologist at Least Once a Year: And more often (every three to six months) if proliferative retinopathy is present. Since the pregnant diabetic is in a high-risk group, she should be checked every other month by the ophthalmologist.

Some questions that many diabetics have for their specialist are these:

Can I wear contact lenses?

Sure, says Dr. L'Esperance, but they should be the soft lens type since diabetes often creates a weak outer layer of cornea tissue and a hard lens is too traumatic for the cornea. And because a diabetic who gets a speck of dust under the lens is more prone to develop a corneal ulcer than a nondiabetic, she should be watched closely by an ophthalmologist—not an optometrist—when she wears contact lenses.

I've heard that Vitamin C can be helpful with eye disease. True?

"Vitamin C has been shown by some studies to be anti capillary-fragility, and if a patient wants to try taking Vitamin C, he should. However, it can throw diabetic control off slightly, so he should check with his regular doctor before starting such a program," says Dr. L'Esperance.

What about exercise?

Excellent, especially the aerobic exercises like swimming. However, if you have retinopathy, do not indulge in contact sports and strenuous, jarring sports that may raise your blood pressure and cause more blow-outs in those tiny, fragile eye vessels. Check with your doctor before any exercise program.

Are chances great that I'll get cataracts in my eyes?

Maybe not great. But Dr. L'Esperance in his book *Diabetic Retinopathy* (with Dr. William A. James, Jr.) says: "the incidence and progression of adult senile cataracts increase in diabetic patients." These cataracts are part of everybody's normal aging process. There's another kind of cataract known as the snowflake metabolic variety that appears in juvenile diabetics and is characterized by chalky white cortical deposits—thus the name, "snowflake."

Kidneys: Diabetic Nephropathy

If the heart is a pump, the kidneys are filters. In healthy adults, each of two kidneys about the size of Idaho potatoes cleanses the blood of waste products, which include chemicals and excess water. As the blood flows through the kidneys, tiny filters catch these waste products and pass them out of the body in about a quart or more of urine a day. The kidneys also work to retain the necessary red and white blood cells and certain vital proteins.

But when diabetes is present, infections, hardening of the small kidney arteries, and damage to the filtering apparatus of the kidney (the glomeruli) can all occur. When any of these things happens, the patient has *diabetic nephropathy.* It doesn't happen overnight. If you've had the disease a long time and it's been in poor control, first, protein in the form of albumin, which the kidney usually retains, starts to appear in the urine. Then more and more water is retained; the patient can gain large amounts of weight because of edema, water-logged tissues. Blood pressure can rise and total kidney failure may come about.

Dr. S. Michael Mauer, Professor of Pediatrics at the University of Minnesota and famed in his area of expertise, kidney disease, says that approximately 30 to 40 percent of insulin-dependent diabetics will develop kidney disease serious enough to end up in kidney failure. In a report presented at the eighth annual scientific meeting of the American Society of Transplant Surgeons in June 1982, the statistics quoted were even higher:

"Fifty percent of individuals with Type I juvenile onset of their disease have, at least in the past, developed uremia from diabetic nephropathy."

As with other diseases, diabetes adds to the complications of kidney problems. Diabetic women are especially prone to urinary infections and these can lead to kidney problems. High blood pressure, says Dr. Mauer, is a particular culprit, and diabetics often are plagued with hypertension. During the first stages of the disease, the physician can treat the kidney disease through dietary routines to make up for the protein being lost and to cope with the lessened ability of the kidneys to excrete wastes. But as the disease progresses, alternate and more drastic measure have to be considered. Dr. Mauer suggests that there are three approaches to dealing with kidney failure:

1. The first approach is to do nothing. As you would expect, that leads to death.

2. The second approach is some form of *dialysis,* the system of attaching a person's blood system to an artificial kidney. One is linked up to a machine for several hours three or four times a week and his blood is taken out of his body, passed through the artificial kidney, cleansed of wastes, then returned to the body in a single continuous circuit. It's painless and it's boring, but it's a lifesaver.

Many patients now have a set-up in their own homes for kidney dialysis, which, incidentally, is subsidized by the government. Others go to a hospital for the procedure. And now, says Dr. Mauer, there's an alternative approach to dialysis known as *peritoneal dialysis.* Researchers at Toronto Western Hospital have developed a new blood-filtering system that uses a patient's internal membranes to screen his blood as he goes through his day. It's called CAPD (Continuous Ambulatory Peritoneal Dialysis). The patient has a catheter installed in his abdomen and attaches a bag, worn externally, to the catheter. The blood is purified by the peritoneum, and because the patient himself can change the fluid, he is freed from the time-consuming ordeal of being hooked to a machine several times a week.

This procedure was originally very difficult to apply to diabetic patients, but more and more success with it is being reported. Dr. Dimitrios Oreopoulos of Toronto Western Hospital, who directed a study of the system, says that the method might well become the treatment of choice for diabetics who need dialysis.

3. The third approach to kidney failure is *transplantation.* Dr. Mauer reports that improved technology, more careful donor selection, better drugs to prevent rejection, and finer surgical techniques have led to steady and consistent improvement in the field. In a recent (June 1982) report to

the American Society of Transplant Surgeons, Dr. David E. R. Sutherland of the University of Minnesota Medical School and his colleagues reported that survival rates in kidney transplants of uremic diabetics came reasonably close (a ratio of 4 to 6) to kidney transplants in non-diabetic patients. This means that the added risk of being a diabetic to transplanted kidney recipients has been shrinking.

Even more interesting, in the same report, was the startling news that the survival rates of diabetics receiving kidney transplants *exceeded* that of uremic diabetics maintained solely on dialysis. And an added plus: in an analysis of diabetic patients who had kidney transplants, 97 percent also had retinopathy. After the transplant, says Dr. Sutherland, the impaired vision of many of these patients improved.

There are about five thousand kidney transplants done each year in the United States. With increased technology, more and more of these appear to be wonderfully successful

According to Dr. Eli A. Friedman, chief of the Renal Diseases Division at Downstate Medical Center in Brooklyn, New York, at least two out of three diabetic kidney recipients will be alive and will have functioning kidneys at least three years after surgery, if they receive a transplant from a living related donor. And when the transplant comes from someone who recently died, about half of the recipients will continue to have a functioning kidney for at least three years. This is extraordinary when one considers that just eight years ago, virtually no diabetics had successful kidney transplants. Dr. Friedman reports that an increasing number of kidney recipients have lived beyond ten years with their transplanted kidneys and the longest-lived kidney recipient has just passed a sixteen-year mark. "There is no question in my mind," says Dr. Friedman, "that for the patient requiring intervention because of uremia, if the full team required to sustain the diabetic is present, a renal transplant is the way to go. What's more, because of the new drug cyclosporine, with its anti-rejection qualities, it will be possible to perform these transplants with a minimum of or no steroids: since steroids are what upsets the glucose balance in transplanted diabetics, this is good news, indeed." So progress is being made in the field. The very best thing a diabetic patient can do, however, is to try to prevent the disease from developing in the first place, and certainly from progressing quickly. Dr. Mauer says there's real evidence, for the first time, on this subject. First and foremost, researchers from Denmark have shown that *hypertension* very markedly accelerates the rate at which the diabetic patient loses kidney function. Blood pressure should be brought under control so that any patient whose pressure is in excess of 140/90 ought to make sure his physician gives him any number of drugs and other treatments that are currently available to bring it down. And second, says Dr. Mauer, animal and some preliminary human studies have showed that "improving the control of the diabetic state—and the bottom line here is normalizing blood sugar—would slow down, arrest, or even circumvent damage to the kidney and other organs as well."

Pancreas

Throughout the world, reports Dr. David Sutherland, there have been only 223 pancreas transplants, the first of which took place in 1966. One hundred twelve of those operations have been performed within the last two years—more than half the total number of transplants ever made. Since 1977, 154 people have received pancreas transplants, and of those, 106 (69 percent) are reported to be still alive. Not a bad average, at all.

Dr. Sutherland reports some further news. In July 1978, the University of Minnesota, long a pioneer in the field, began a series of pancreas transplants in fifty patients. As of August 1982, forty-one of the fifty patients were still alive—the longest for 4.1 years after transplantation. Seventeen of those recipients were shown to be insulin independent (in essence, cured of diabetes), with normal or nearly normal glucose tolerance levels.

Now, while those numbers really represent a drop in the bucket when compared to the numbers of insulin-dependent people suffering from problems due to a pancreas that doesn't function properly, they are cause for "renewed interest" by researchers and surgeons, says Dr. Sutherland.* "Although the success rate is still relatively low, the mortality and morbidity is much lower than in previous years and long term graft function has been sustained in several patients."

It's too early to tell definitively, says the doctor, but a drug with anti-rejection qualities called cyclosporine may have improved the results of pancreas transplantation. Because the drug has potential side effects, its use is currently restricted to patients who have very serious complications from diabetes.

So, the ultimate cure for diabetes—pancreas transplants—has a long way to go before being perfected for general public use. The problems of rejection are being gained on by today's surgeons and researchers, but realistically considered, the art of pancreas transplantation is still quite experimental. It is greatly encouraging to know that scientists are working in increasingly successful ways to find the answers.

Nerves: Diabetic Neuropathy

One of the most common complications of diabetes is damage to the peripheral nerves that run throughout the body connecting the spinal cord to

* *Transplantation Proceedings,* 15:1 (March 1983).

muscles, skin, blood vessels, and all the other organs. Think of the nerve as an electric light cord with its insulation frayed or destroyed and the raw wire, or nerve, exposed. When that nerve is damaged, it hurts because it's not protected.

The longest nerves are the most vulnerable, says Dr. Fred W. Whitehouse, head of the Division of Metabolic Disease at the Henry Ford Hospital in Detroit, Michigan, and so legs and feet are most often the extremities that are involved, with arms and hands coming in for a close second. Symptoms can range all the way from a loss of feeling, a tingling sensation ("My feet feel as though they fell asleep," is a common complaint) to burning, darting, or aching pains. This is called *peripheral neuropathy*; it involves voluntary nerves to the arms, legs, and muscles and it's often worse at night. When neuropathy strikes involuntary nerve areas in the gastrointestinal tract, the bladder, the penis, and other body organs, it's known as *autonomic neuropathy*. Here the symptoms may be impotence in males, diarrhea, abnormal sweating, poor emptying of the bladder or stomach, and others.

When pain is present, "the simple pain relievers like Darvon or aspirin are the best," says Dr. Whitehouse. "They're given in place of the stronger, narcotic drugs in the hope that after six to twenty-four months of good blood sugar control, the patient's neuropathy will lessen in severity. Although the evidence is paltry on this subject, perhaps the nerves do regenerate themselves or become less damaged.

"Drugs that are similar to antidepressants, like Elavil, Sinequan, or, for sharp, shooting pains, Tegretol, are frequently prescribed," says Dr. Whitehouse. "Patients with intestinal neuropathy find that anti-diarrhea medications like Lomotil work well. Constipation usually responds to mild laxatives and stool softeners."

Although there are some specific remedies and palliatives for neuropathic problems, "the sine qua non of neuropathy is getting that blood sugar under control."

Dr. Daniel Porte, a specialist in the problems of neuropathy who works at the University of Washington in Seattle, Washington, agrees.

"Neuropathy is basically a preventative problem," he says, "which very likely relates to the quality of blood sugar control and to the duration of the diabetes. So many drugs are touted publicly to be panaceas and they are not. For instance: the dietary nutrient known as myoinositol has been used experimentally under very limited conditions, and under these conditions seems to have some beneficial effect on neuropathic complications. In high concentrations, though, it's a toxic compound and should never be bought and used off the shelf as you can find it in health food stores."

Many patients with neuropathic problems tend to overload their diets with particular foods they've "heard" can be helpful.

"A big mistake," comments Dr. Porte. "Patients should never be involved in self-prescribing for their neuropathy. Bizarre diets where patients consume large amounts of food they've heard is 'good for them,' and ignore other nutritional needs in the process, can be hazardous."

Are there any new drugs that can be used to treat diabetic neuropathy? There is one interesting drug not yet in the marketplace, says Dr. Porte. Aldose reductase is the enzyme that's responsible for the formation of certain cataracts in the eye. Recent evidence has shown that aldose reductase may also be involved in diabetic neuropathy in which a decreased velocity of impulse transmission exists in the motor and sensory nerves. A new drug called sorbinil has been shown to be effective for some patients in improving their motor and sensory nerve conduction velocity. But, cautions Dr. Porte, sorbinil is still involved in Federal Drug Administration clinical trials and won't be available for a while.

Other autonomic neuropathies are treated with specific therapies. Your doctor can medically empty your stomach with a new drug called Reglan (metaclopramide) if you have this gastrointestinal problem. Impotence can sometimes be treated in a variety of ways, including penile transplants. An interesting word about the latter comes from Dr. Richard Bernstein, author of *Diabetes: The Glucograf Method for Normalizing Blood Sugar.* He writes to say that one of the most feared diabetic complications is neuropathic impotence; yet the lack of ability to achieve erection may not be a true neuropathic problem at all but simply the result of having hypoglycemia (low blood sugar) at "the wrong time." Hypoglycemia "is not the only cause of sexual dysfunction, but for insulin users, it's the most common." Dr. Bernstein notes that many men write to him wanting to know if they can get rid of their penile transplants when they discover they're not suffering from neuropathic penile problems but too many blood sugar episodes.

The one comforting thought about diabetic neuropathy is that if the pain waxes, as time progresses it also usually wanes. It seems endless, it tries your courage as well as your patience—but it does seem to abate eventually, leaving numbness in the involved areas. There is very little specific therapy for neuropathy. This is one of the reasons that the JDF works so singlemindedly toward helping research scientists to find the answers.

Cardiovascular Disease

Nobody really knows what the effects of diabetes are on cardiovascular disease, but we do know that arteriosclerotic heart disease is the greatest single cause of death in the United States, and the National Institutes of

Health estimates that diabetics are twice as prone to coronary heart disease, twice as prone to stroke, and five times as prone to arterial disease of the limbs as non-diabetics. Moreover, about 75 percent of deaths among diabetics are due to cardiovascular diseases, as opposed to 50 percent of the deaths in the general population. So diabetes is really bad news for health of the heart and of the vessels through which blood and its fuel reach every part of the body.

Diabetics have a special problem: a tendency toward *hyperlipidemia.* This is a condition in which too many lipids (blood fats) tend to circulate in the bloodstream, instead of being stored, which leads to an accumulation of fatty deposits on blood vessel walls. When these walls thicken from the fat substances, blood cannot flow through easily. Insulin deficiencies in diabetics may also bring about changes in the metabolism of vascular tissue. High blood pressure, a common complaint of diabetics, puts extra strain on all the blood vessels, including the heart. And obesity, which brings about stress because of the added blood supply needed to fuel the extra fat tissues, is also a problem for many diabetics—although maturity-onset diabetics seem to be more involved with problems of obesity than insulin-dependent diabetics.

Are diabetics helpless when it comes to self-care and cardiovascular problems? Most assuredly not.

Dr. Antonio Gotto, chairman of Internal Medicine at the Baylor College of Medicine, Methodist Hospital, in Houston, Texas, says there are three major risk factors to avoid. And they are the very same risk factors that anyone who does not have diabetes might well try to consider if he is to help himself avoid arteriosclerosis. They are:

—*Smoking:* Don't do it! Ample evidence shows that tobacco has a distinctly poor effect on blood vessels, which constrict from arterial spasms with each inhalation.

—*High Blood Pressure:* Get it down—your doctor will tell you how! Dr. Gotto says that the diabetic patient is particularly susceptible to small vessel disease in the eye and kidney because of elevated blood pressure.

—*High Fat Diets:* Avoid them! Saturated fats tend to elevate plasma-cholesterol, bad news for diabetics—and everyone else in the world.

Aside from avoiding these three risk factors, exercise appropriate for the individual has a *very* beneficial effect on glucose metabolism, decreases insulin requirements, and lowers cholesterol levels. Dr. Charles Peterson and Dr. Anthony Cerami of the Rockefeller Institute in New York, as mentioned earlier in this book, are conducting work on exercise to see what value it can be to diabetics. High-density lipoproteins in the blood sugar appear to carry fat lipids out of the cells, and exercise tends to raise the number of high-density lipoproteins in the body; therefore, the more HDLs (high-density lipoproteins) you have, the less chance there is of developing hardening of the arteries, say the doctors. Aerobic exercises—like walking briskly, running, or swimming—that lower cholesterol and triglyceride (high blood fats), condition the heart, lungs, and blood vessels, and increase the body's ability to utilize its oxygen intake are particularly good ... if your doctor recommends them. Be sure that you have an exercise program tailormade for you from an expert who is thoroughly familiar with diabetes management.

Amputation

It's a very frightening word, but since 20 to 40 percent of the diabetic population is more liable to develop gangrene than the non-diabetic population, it's also a fact of life to be considered. Amputations *are* some of the "worst that can happen," but the chances of avoiding this disaster are much brighter than ever before.

What causes the complications that can lead to amputation? Our legs, feet, arms, and hands are absolutely dependent on a steady and nourishing flow of blood. When that flow is interrupted because of progressive vascular disease, a complication of diabetes, the result is tissue death—or gangrene. And when the gangrene is bad enough, amputation is required.

Dr. Charles R. Shuman, Professor of Medicine at Temple University School of Medicine in Philadelphia, says there are three specific indications for amputation. They are the presence of severe pain; uncontrollable infection; and/or uncontrollable diabetes—all associated with gangrene. If the gangrene is "dry" (the absence of infection) and there are some small blood vessels that can carry even just a little bit of blood through to the limbs, the disease may progress more slowly and postpone the amputation that will eventually be necessary.

What can be done? Well, in the first place, too many uninformed doctors recommend vaso-dilator drugs, which many non-diabetic patients with arteriosclerosis take to help increase blood flow. In the diabetic patient, says Dr. Shuman, the vaso-dilators are of very little use; and in some cases, drugs like propanolol (inderal) can actually decrease the flow and aggravate the process causing tissue death. What has been quite effective generally is a bypass operation known as a *saphenous vein graft*. This surgical procedure, when successful, has reduced the frequency of gangrene and has, in the presence of gangrene, "allowed us to get away with much more peripheral amputation—a toe rather than a leg—for example."

Other surgical procedures include *balloon angioplasty*, a radiological technique by which a catheter is passed into a narrowed artery: if the narrowing is localized, a balloon at the end of the catheter can widen the artery. Unfortunately, vascular disease in diabetics is often too widespread for this procedure to be frequently employed. Still another, but again not often successful surgical procedure that may be tried is a *lumbar sympathectomy*. This involves removing the nerves that constrict the blood vessels.

The very best approach to deter or hopefully avoid the progressive vascular disease that leads to amputation, says Dr. Shuman, "is a lifestyle which includes

- the control of serum lipids (fatty substances in the blood)
- the very good control of blood sugar
- adequate exercise
- and, most strenuously, the avoidance of smoking."

Skin Problems

The skin is the largest body organ, and if diabetics are particularly susceptible to problems in other organs, the skin is no exception. Poorly controlled blood sugar often leads to very dry skin, which is tempting to scratch, thereby opening your skin up, literally, to bacterial infections.

A common skin condition is known as *diabetic dermopathy*, or "shin spots," says Dr. Irwin Braverman, Professor of Dermatology at the Yale University School of Medicine in New Haven. "The patient looks as if he's struck his shins, repeatedly, but there's no history of trauma." They're not painful and there's no real cure for them.

With poor blood sugar control come "xanthomas." These are hard, bumpy eruptions that appear on the buttocks, knees, and elbows, and disappear when the blood sugar is more stabilized.

Less common are small blisters that start up on hands and feet, says Dr. Braverman, often growing to 4 or 5 inches in diameter. They take three to six weeks to heal and tend to reoccur.

One of the most common and also annoying skin conditions is known as *necrobiosis lipoidica diabeticorum* (NLD); it is characterized by discolored and dimpled skin in which the layers of fat directly underneath have disappeared. This is not dangerous but cosmetically disturbing because it appears first as a pink discoloration, then as shiny and tight lesions. Ointments are usually not useful except for some improvement being noted from cortisone ointments; fine needle injections of cortisone are also used with some success, says a report from the Joslin Institute.

Fungal infections in diabetes are often caused by the yeastlike fungus monilia, says Dr. J. E. Jelinek, Clinical Professor of Dermatology at the New York University Medical School in New York. They usually appear as itchy rashes of moist red areas, surrounded by tiny blisters and scales, in the folds of the skin that tend to be warm and moist—armpits, groins, under breasts, in the margins of the nails, between fingers or toes, in the corners of the mouth, and under the foreskin of uncircumsized males. Poor control is a likely culprit of cause. Keeping groin and feet dry with unscented talcum powder helps prevent these fungal infections so common in diabetes, and drying the hands often is important for people like homemakers, bartenders, and waiters whose hands are frequently wet. Yeast infections are treated with a prescription from your doctor for an appropriate medication. Note: compresses of half a tablespoon of vinegar to a quart of tap water may give some relief, says Dr. Jelinek.

Athlete's foot, not seen more often in diabetics than non-diabetics, can lead to a bacterial infection. It should be cleared up quickly with Tinactin (available without prescription) in lotion, cream, or powder form, or Desenex, another over-the-counter preparation.

Perhaps the most common skin problem diabetics have is known as hypertrophy or *insulin atrophy*. In the sites where insulin injections are frequently given comes a loss of fatty tissue, creating deep hollows. Luckily, with the purer insulins, these "dented" areas are becoming less common. The remedy is to use varied sites for injection, giving the dents time to fill in again—as they usually do. Room-temperature insulin is usually helpful in bypassing the depressions.

General skin care consists of not allowing the skin to become dehydrated and dried out ... a condition of poor control. Some suggestions to avoid this follow:

—Avoid overlogging with too much showering and bathing, especially in cold weather. Use superfatted soaps.

—Protect your skin with dry-skin creams or ointments. After a bath, and before sleep at night, it's a good idea to leave the skin just slightly moist and then apply a thin layer of Vaseline. This protects it and keeps moisture sealed in for the night.

—Dry, itchy skin that's been cracked open from scratching or other abuse should be treated with anything that seems to help: topical steroids, emollients, or whatever your dermatologist thinks is beneficial. The important thing is not to allow that skin to stay open to bacterial invasion.

WHAT'S NEW IN AVAILABLE TREATMENTS

Home Blood Glucose Monitoring

We've really gone into this fully in the Sugar Babies chapter, so just a few more words on home monitoring of blood. The most exciting advance in diabetes management during this century has been the advent of home blood glucose monitoring instead of urine testing. This form of control allows one to respond immediately to the exact, current level of sugar in the blood rather than guessing or estimating from urine tests, "feelings," or waiting until the doctor's blood test comes through. And yet, unbelievably, most people still rely on measuring urine sugar to determine how much insulin, diet, and exercise they should take. How come? We can't understand it. What's more, and worse, we can't understand the hesitance of some doctors to recommend home blood monitoring to their patients. Unless there is some mysterious deeply held phobia of patients to blood monitoring at home, *there can be no good reason for not opting to control one's blood sugar in this accurate way.*

There's another reason, recently brought to our attention by Dr. Richard Bernstein of the Westchester Medical College of Valhalla, New York, for monitoring your own sugar. It makes you feel *psychologically* better. It gives you control. For years, doctors have been telling patients to keep their sugar in control, without teaching them the means to do so accurately. For years they have been telling patients to be "compliant," without telling them how to do it. And for years, says Dr. Bernstein, patients have been feeling stress and depression at their inability to be "good." "Compliance" was virtually impossible with urine testing, "compliance" became a hated word in the diabetes lexicon.

With the exception of one paper written by Dr. Andre Dupois, a psychiatrist at the Cornell University Medical College, together with Drs. Robert Jones and Charles Peterson at Rockefeller University, which stated that self-monitoring of blood glucose led not only to better diabetes control but to improved emotional status, not one research study notes a connection between the mode of medical treatment and the emotional state of patients, says Dr. Bernstein. Yet when people monitor their own blood sugar, it allows them to eliminate anxiety about the questions, "Is my blood glucose too high, am I anxious or hungry, or is my blood glucose too low?" It allows a measure of diabetic control, counteracting the helplessness that many feel when control is out of their hands. One patient told Dr. Bernstein: "For twenty-five years, I felt as if I were on a rudderless ship allowing my body to deteriorate . . . I had also been conditioned to think that this lack of control allowed for a carefree lifestyle in which you 'forgot' about your disease." After learning how to monitor his own blood at home, the patient, for the first time, felt in command of his own life. "Compliance" took on a new meaning.

Monitoring one's own blood lets you be a self-advocate in the finest sense of the word. It gives you responsibility, taking away the father image of the physician who can no longer have any reason to give you the "guilties." When a patient feels better, as he no doubt will with home monitoring, he no longer is at odds with "compliance." How can you be compliant when what they want you to do makes no sense? Adolescents especially, says Dr. Bernstein, "grasp at any opportunity for independence and control of their own ballgames."

The Creation of Human Insulin

This past year has seen a remarkable advance for diabetes: the development of human insulin, not extracted from the human pancreas but produced synthetically in laboratories. Up till now, insulin users have relied on insulin extracted from the pancreases of animals, usually pigs or cows. It worked fairly well and it saved lives, of course; but there have always been at least two problems that plagued the users of animal insulin.

First of all, there were allergies: some diabetics are allergic to animal insulin. Second of all, availability: the supply of insulin is dependent upon the supply of meat animals which, some authorities feel, may someday become scarce. Insulin users don't love the idea of what can happen if these supplies run short—rationed insulin or wildly expensive insulin, in effect, insulin not dependably available. Now, two human insulin–producing techniques have been developed, and when the insulin from these sources becomes proven and available to all, the worries of diabetics all over the world will be over.

One of these new insulins is pioneered by Eli Lilly & Company and utilizes "recombinant DNA" technology.* DNA (deoxyribonucleic acid) carries the genetic information that enables species to reproduce their own kind. It is DNA that ordains whether an organism is a dog, a person, a fish, a virus, or a red tomato. When scientists found out how to recombine genetic material, to synthesize whole molecules from bacteria, says Dr. Gerold Grodsky, Professor of Biochemistry and associate research director of the Metabolic Unit of the University of California in San Francisco, they were able to create synthesis genes to make human insulin. What they had done was splice the genes into an organism known as *E. coli* bacteria, and

*See chart on human insulin in "III. General Information," p. 235.

the bacteria produced human insulin. Clinical trials began; as of March 1982, nine hundred patients were being treated with human insulin therapy.

The insulin created by genetic engineering is an answer to the threat of an insulin shortage and the product is, in every way, identical to human insulin, not the beef or pork insulin that's been in use for almost six decades. There are many intricate processes of recombinant DNA techniques. Researchers at Eli Lilly say that all of them now existing, and those expected to develop, will include these basic steps:

- identifying useful genes
- isolating the genes into a host cell
- reproducing the cell containing the new DNA.

Another technique, pioneered by Novo Industri in Denmark, creates human insulin from biochemically transformed cattle and swine insulin. Molecular modification of animal insulin also produces excellent human insulin, but does not address the problems of future shortages of animal pancreas glands or of allergies to pork- or beef-based insulins.

Dr. Grodsky says it is too soon to know which method of producing human insulin will be best in terms of cost reduction to the diabetic who must purchase it. But the healthy competition between two companies will certainly be very good in holding down the price of all synthesized insulins, says one biochemist who does not wish to be identified. Comments Dr. Grodsky: "The potential of molecular engineering is enormous for researchers and it's just begun to be tapped. Not only does it give us the advantage of being able to create insulin, but it gives us a new way of looking at cells—research that's of inestimable importance to finding a cure for diabetes."

The Insulin Infusion Pump

It has long been a dream of scientists to be able to deliver insulin in much the same way that the human pancreas delivers it, when the person needs it, rather than being tied down to subcutaneous injections. Injections confine their users to certain patterns of exercise, diet, and mealtimes; a continuous delivery system would enable the user to deliver the insulin at the times when his body required it. Well, all the kinks have not been worked out, and as with every new invention, there are its defenders and its critics. But the insulin pump is here, in use, and generating real excitement in the world of scientists and diabetes patients.

Several kinds of pumps have been developed. Most are enclosed in small boxes worn on a belt. The pumps have tiny needles attached to them; these needles are placed under the skin, and sometimes in a vein, depending on the kind of pump. The user, by pushing a button, can give himself a rather continuous trickle of insulin into the bloodstream—with extra dollops before meals—when he needs it. This is called "an open loop system" because it is necessary for the patient to program the times and amounts of insulin to be delivered into his system.

Another system of delivery is the "closed loop" system, which uses an implantable sensor that reads blood sugar levels, then sends a message to a computer that activates the pump to release as much insulin as the patient needs—without the patient himself doing anything. As we go to press, researchers at the University of Minnesota report success with pumps about the size of hockey pucks, implanted under the skin in several body locations; these pumps deliver continuous drips of insulin into the blood and have worked continuously for up to a year, so far. They can be refilled without being removed. Patients report them as being "forgettable—they allow a more normal lifestyle," according to the researchers in an article printed in the *New England Journal of Medicine.* The team, headed by Dr. Henry Buchwald, says that almost all the problems run into by wearers of external pumps can be avoided by putting the pumps into the skin.

The pumps still come under the heading of experimental research because there are many problems to be worked out. For instance, Dr. Gerold Grodsky brings up the uncomfortable point that some patients who have been on the pump for a year seem to be getting more severe eye disease than should be expected. "Perhaps the pump, as it's presented now, overcontrols; perhaps it forces a person to go too quickly from bad control to good; or perhaps the sites of injection have to be reconsidered (the pumps now place insulin either under the skin or into the body cavity, while the normal pancreas puts insulin into a portal vein which goes directly to the liver). Whether it's one thing or another, we know the pumps are still quite crude, and we now we have to learn quite a lot about how to refine them."

Still, the pumps, crude as they are, are proving an important advance in diabetic progress. Experiments with pregnant women who are placed on the pump in the first critical months of pregnancy, and tests with adolescents who traditionally have wide swings in blood sugar, have proved happily successful in normalizing blood sugar better than ever before. Moreover, the pumps, because they allow for stability in blood sugar, also encourage more steady, more normal hormone levels.

Quite important and interesting has been patient response:

"They're great—you don't have to be tied down to meals at specific hours!"

"You don't always have to be looking for a bathroom to give yourself a shot in privacy."

"You don't have to carry syringes and insulin around, wherever you go, any more."

"I had such problems with my first pregnancy—this one is progressing so smoothly!"

Dr. William V. Tamborlane, Jr., at the Yale University School of Medicine, part of a team that has led the fight for the insulin pump research, says that pump treatment should be limited to doctors who are trained in its use. He cautions also that we do not know whether long-term pump use will have any negative effects and we do not yet know whether the pump will definitely prevent complications. Therefore, "Carefully controlled, step-by-step use of this new technology [is recommended] . . . rather than its premature application on a large scale."

So more testing is in the cards to work out some of the pump's problems. These include mechanical pump failure, awkward pump size, and delivery that is not always reliable. But the implications of this invention are profound, offering great hope for better control and ease of living to the diabetic.

Pregnancy and Fetal Development

One of the areas of diabetic research that has shown the most significant advances has been that of childbirth. Traditionally, infants of mothers with diabetes have significantly greater risk of mortality, respiratory distress, prematurity, and other serious problems. The diabetic woman having a baby in 1983 has lucked out. Careful metabolic regulation for almost every insulin-dependent diabetic woman is a reality now that the insulin pump and multiple insulin injections are prescribed by doctors along with the all-important availability of home blood testing. Specific tests and hormone evaluations have hugely improved the picture of childbirth. According to a report of the National Diabetes Advisory Board, "except for congenital anomalies and some neonatal morbidity," diabetic mothers have almost the same chance of producing a healthy baby as non-diabetic mothers.

The absolutely essential difference has been this: it requires a specialist, consummately trained in the problems that women with diabetes have during pregnancy, to oversee the preparation before conception, the pregnancy, and the birth of a baby to a diabetic mother. Any woman not seeking out such a specialist when she plans to have a baby is cutting her chances for a successful pregnancy greatly, says Dr. Lester Salans, Director of the National Institute of Arthritis, Diabetes, and Digestive and Kidney

Diseases, in Bethesda, Md. "The only thing that has not been influenced [by the new technology] is the frequency of congenital malformations in infants born to diabetic mothers. That may be because we are not intervening soon enough in the course of a pregnancy." Dr. Steven Gabbe, the obstetrician at Children's Hospital in Philadelphia who specializes in diabetic pregnancies, agrees, suggesting that the months *before* conception are the optimum time for a diabetic woman to see an expert. He/she can tell you how best to prepare your body for pregnancy even before a fetus takes up residence.

The National Diabetes Research Interchange (NDRI)

QUESTION: *What's worth more than gold and harder to get?*
ANSWER: Human tissues for research.

It's one thing to make great advances in the world of mice colonies; it's quite another to find out how such research applies to human beings. In order to develop new treatments, and eventually a cure for diabetes, it is vital to have human tissues available for scientific research. But until last year, such tissues were either carelessly discarded or impossible to obtain for other reasons, and scientists were often stymied in their efforts. It became clear that founding the Juvenile Diabetes Foundation was just a beginning. There would also have to be an organization to procure, preserve, and deliver the tissues and human organs so invaluable in discovering the pathogenesis and treatment of diabetic complications.

Early in 1980, Lee was proud and thrilled to be able to witness the birth of her new baby, The National Diabetes Research Interchange, established by a grant from the Pew Memorial Trust. NDRI—a unique, computerized organization—takes it upon itself to find and deliver to scientists everything from the umbilical cord from a Caesarean section to an "unplaceable" kidney from a transplant program. This special program, an affiliate of JDF, has been nationally acclaimed as a major boon to the future of diabetes research. In its first year, it delivered over one thousand tissue samples to research laboratories to provide clues to a cure.

Within hours of first notification, donated tissues and organs (eyes, pancreas, etc.) are rushed to the NDRI's laboratory facilities, where they're preserved and prepared for shipping to diabetes researchers nationwide. And "if the NDRI program is successful," comments Dr. Salans, "it can serve as a very important model for other diseases."

THE CRYSTAL BALL ... WHAT'S AHEAD IN RESEARCH?

What's Ahead in Eye Research?

Dr. Robert Frank, an ophthalmologist at the Kresge Eye Institute of the Wayne State School of Medicine in Detroit, is studying blood vessels in order to find the causes of diabetic retinopathy. He and his co-workers have demonstrated the ability to grow whole retinal vessel mounts in a type of tissue culture preparation, in order "to investigate their biochemistry and examine their anatomical structure, particularly as it may be modified by diabetes ... in this way we may be able to alleviate the complications of diabetes."

Certain biochemical mechanisms may also be responsible for the first changes of diabetic retinopathy. Among them is the enzyme known as aldose reductase, which is known to be responsible for cataracts in young diabetics. Dr. Kenneth Gabbay, director of the Children's Hospital Medical Center in Boston and Associate Professor of Medicine at Harvard Medical School, says that "aldose reductase converts glucose and other sugars into sugar alcohols called sorbitol, which are metabolized very slowly once they are formed inside cells. As their concentrations increase, they cause swelling and permanent damage to the cells." When this occurs in the eye lens, cataracts result. Experimental evidence with animals has shown that inhibitors of the enzyme can block it, and by preventing the glucose from converting to sorbitol, can also prevent cataract formation in the eye. Ongoing research will hopefully show that aldose reductase inhibitors will work to prevent cataracts in humans.

—Dr. Alan Shabo at the University of California at Los Angeles is working on immunological studies in animals to question the role that a possible sensitization to insulin may be involved in retinopathy.

—Dr. Ronald Engerman of the University of Wisconsin is studying the role that strict blood sugar control plays in retinopathy. He's recently discovered that frequent insulin injections, better control, and administration of the chemical Alloxan have reduced the severity of diabetic retinopathy in laboratory animals.

—Dr. Judah Folkman and co-workers at Boston Children's Hospital are working on discovering factors in the retina that stimulate new blood vessel growth and proliferation.

—Recent studies have shown that plain old aspirin may help to prevent retinopathy and slow its progression, once it's contracted, and the National Eye Institute in Maryland is currently examining this problem.

So, rest assured that all kinds of research is going on to ensure that eye problems from diabetes will, one day, be a thing of the past. Some of the finest scientists in the most prestigious institutions all over the world are committed to finding a preventative and ultimately a cure for diabetic retinopathy.

What's Ahead in Pancreas Transplants?

When doctors achieved the first successful kidney transplants, hope for helping diabetics through pancreas transplants grew. The major problem in any kind of transplantation has always been immunologic rejection; the body tends to reject what's foreign to it. Drug treatment, especially with steroids, often creates other problems, including an acceleration of kidney damage that is particularly dangerous for diabetic patients. Dr. David Sutherland of the University of Minnesota Medical School says that since much of pancreas transplantation should take place *before* complications become too severe, methods are being studied to identify patients who are at high risk of developing disastrous complications. One of the "predictive" features is the tendency of some children to have limited joint mobility in childhood. Their fingers seem stiffer than those of other children and may foretell diabetes patients who will have difficulty controlling their blood sugar.

Other studies will focus on the procurement of pancreases for diabetic patients who could potentially benefit from pancreas transplantation. "There is no inherent reason," says Dr. Sutherland, "why procurement of pancreases should be any different from procurement of kidneys for transplantation."

The all-important study of new drugs to halt rejection will be continued on a increased scale, particularly investigation of the drug cyclosporine, which has had some success in smaller studies.

Techniques of transplantation will be studied more closely in the next few years. For instance, it's recently been found, reports Dr. Sutherland, that most recipients of pancreas transplants have also had kidney transplants. It appears that patient survival is higher when a kidney is transplanted first, and then followed by a pancreas, rather than a simultaneous pancreas-kidney transplant.

Although there's a long road to go, "the potential for application of pancreas transplantation probably exceeds that of the liver and may approach that of the kidney."

Islet Cell Transplants

Since the islets of Langerhans contain the pancreas's insulin-producing beta cells, finding a way to transplant these islets to humans would be of inestimable value. The scientist most responsible for much of the progress in this field has been Dr. Paul E. Lacy who, with his team at the Washington University School of Medicine, two years ago developed a procedure for the successful transplantation of clusters of the insulin-producing cells, from one animal species to another. The investigators further showed that the beta cells within the islets, taken from healthy rats, could reverse diabetes in the diabetic mice that received the transplants.

It is very difficult to extract useful quantities of islet cells from the human pancreas, so other sources are needed. Islet cells transplants in experimental animals of different strains have always been impeded by the problem of immune rejection, so Dr. Lacy and his colleagues' success has enormous implications in the world of transplants of every sort, including heart, kidney, and so on. Now, Dr. Lacy reports, the research has proceeded to trying the procedures in dogs and monkeys. And if they are successful there, the approaches will be attempted in man.

"I can't give you a timetable on that," Dr. Lacy says. "I've learned that sometimes when I think all is going well, I hit a stumbling block, and then it's back to the drawing board for another two years. But there is surely cause for hope and optimism. We're on the right track, having come farther in experimentation than ever before. If we can remove the white blood cells that say to the body, 'Hey, you've got foreign tissue to get rid of,' we can eliminate that which contaminates the transplant."

There are many problems, of course, and while there is great excitement in the air with Dr. Lacy's work, he cautions against expecting that his animal research will be immediately applicable to humans. Some problems include finding out whether islet transplants from one species to another will function well over long periods of time. It also will be critical to find out the number of islet cells needed to maintain normal blood sugar levels. Still another problems in finding a way to have the transplant take without using immunity-suppressing drugs that seriously weaken a patient's immunity system, making her vulnerable to life-threatening infections. And further research is needed to determine the best site for these islet implantations to achieve optimal blood glucose control, as well as a way to remove the islets if an adverse reaction should occur.

Work goes on in the study of islet cell transplants. It's exhilarating to follow because when the problems have been solved, this is the scientific advance that does not mean treatment or slowing down of diabetes; it means cure.

What's Ahead in Research into Kidney Complications?

Kidney transplants seem to have a high evidence of success and new procedures are being refined daily, says Dr. S. Michael Mauer, even though there have been no revolutionary breakthroughs. The process is more evolutionary; and because of improved ways to control blood sugar, for one thing, the grafts are functioning better and better. Studies in normalization of blood glucose and in islet cell transplantation continue to demonstrate that these two factors can eventually reverse and prevent kidney damage in humans.

Scientists have also been studying the relationship of hormonal and other substances to the development of diabetic nephropathy, as well as the biochemistry of the membranes of the kidney, says a report from the National Diabetes Advisory Board, in an effort to discover how to prevent the thickening that occurs so characteristically in diabetes.

The National Institutes of Health reports preliminary investigations to show that changes in the pattern of urinary excretion of certain enzymes may be an early, sensitive sign of kidney disease in diabetic patients. Pinpointing the disease at an early stage may help enormously in its treatment, say the researchers.

Dr. Eli Friedman, specialist in kidney transplants in New York, says the "biopsies of kidneys that have been transplanted into diabetics show the recurrence, after about three years, of the same process that destroyed the person's own kidneys. So far, although we have evidence that the diabetic changes in the transplants become more pronounced after five years, we have no indication that the kidney's function is impaired. This makes sense. If it took twenty years for diabetes to cause kidney failure in the first place, it will probably take another twenty for the transplant to fail." Dr. Friedman predicts that in ten or twenty years, our methods of blood glucose control may be so improved that we'll be able to arrest such destruction in transplants.

What's Ahead in Research into Neuropathy?

Dr. Daniel Porte says that research is being conducted on sorbitol-blocking drugs. The enzyme aldose reductase turns high glucose into fructose and then into sorbitol, a sugar that causes tissues to be waterlogged and unable to metabolize properly. The peripheral nerves in this "sorbitol pathway" also can build up a sorbitol accumulation—a neuropathic complication that can create pain and interfere with the nerves' ability to conduct messages.

Further, the National Diabetes Advisory Board reports that scientists are studying the role that various biochemical substances play in neuropathic disorders, particularly the 41st amino acid polypeptide known as corticotropin releasing factor. It may be involved in stress-induced bodily responses like high blood sugar which, in turn, are very damaging to the body's nerves.

The National Institute of Neurological and Communicative Disorders and Stroke (NINCDS) has established a peripheral neuropathy clinical research center at the Mayo Foundation. Researchers are examining the supposed accumulation of alcohol sugars to damaged nerve fibers. They are also examining the question of whether the dietary nutrient myoinositol is, in diabetes, decreased in peripheral neurons. NINCDS research is delving into non-hormonal blood factors, lipoproteins, cholesterol, and triglycerides, too, to see how they affect peripheral neuropathy.

What's Ahead in Research into Cardiovascular Complications?

Dr. Antonio Gotto reports much research going on at the cellular level. The question scientists are currently working to answer is: How can we protect cells in the arterial walls from developing arteriosclerosis?

Studies are being conducted to discover what, if any, relationship an excess of insulin adds to the already known risk factors of cardiovascular disease. Other studies are evaluating the value certain fibers like bran have in lowering blood cholesterol. Dr. Gotto says that in experiments requiring a highly specialized diet of 30 to 40 grams of daily fiber (more than a little All-Bran for breakfast), some encouraging results have been shown.

The ubiquitous drug aspirin is also being studied to see what its anticlotting effect has been on vascular disease. Research has shown that aspirin may sometimes lower blood sugar and help prevent eye changes. But check with your own doctor before you supplement your diet with aspirin: it *could* have negative results on diabetes management.

Low cholesterol diets are being closely watched to see if they really have an effect on blood serum. Research has shown that it is generally advantageous to follow a diet high in the polyunsaturated fats that are derived from vegetable rather than animal origin. According to Dr. Stuart Soeldner, Associate Professor of Medicine at Peter Bent Brigham Hospital, Harvard Medical School, and an associate at the Joslin Diabetes Foundation in Boston, a diet low in cholesterol and saturated fats, together with insulin control of blood glucose, has been more effective than a conventional diabetic diet in reducing the incidence of hyperlipoproteinemia (an excess of proteins and fats in the blood) in children with insulin-dependent diabetes.

The study of platelets (cellular components of the coagulation system) is an area of research currently getting much attention. Platelets adhering and clumping together in the blood vessel walls may take part in the building up of arteriosclerotic deposits, causing clots and blockage of blood flow to toes and feet. Dr. Marvin E. Levin, associate director of the Metabolism Clinic at the Washington University School of Medicine in St. Louis, says early research has shown that injections of prostacyclin (a substance that prevents platelets from sticking together) may improve circulation through already narrowed vessels.

Meanwhile vascular surgeons are steadily improving new techniques to replace the damaged arteries of diabetes patients who have had poorly controlled blood sugar for long years. These operations are performed to protect the heart (coronary bypasses) feet and leg (femoral bypasses) and brain (carotid bypasses) so that the rate of heart attacks, insufficiency of circulation in the feet and legs, and stroke in patients with diabetes may all be lowered.

Dr. Gotto suggests that lowering blood sugar may well help avoid cardiovascular complications, but he cautions that not enough data are available to prove that definitively. The results of a new, large-scale study to determine the relationship between blood glucose control and complications (to be discussed at the end of this chapter) will give us the answer eagerly sought by so many.

One of the most important advances in diabetes detection and control of blood sugar has been the development of the Hemoglobin A1c Test. Hemoglobin A1c is hemoglobin with glucose attached to it. Normally Hemoglobin A1c comprises less than 6 percent of your total hemoglobin, but persistently high blood sugar levels increase it. When your physician takes a simple Hemoglobin A1c Test, he can determine how well your body has controlled its blood glucose over approximately three months. The test is unaffected by the food you ate (or didn't eat) or the exercise or stress you've had just before you took the test, so you can't fool it and you can't change results as you can with a regular blood sugar test. A normal level ranges between 4 to 7 percent.

This test should be done regularly to assess your overall blood sugar control (regularly means at least every six months). If control is definitely proven to have positive effects on cardiovascular complications, the Hemoglobin A1c Test will be an invaluable aid to finding that control.

Genetic Markers

If you and your husband are flaming redheads, chances are that when you have a baby, your genes will produce another redhead for you. That's heredity. Researchers and families of diabetics have long suspected that heredity must also have something to say about who gets diabetes and who doesn't. But *which* are the genes that might make a person susceptible to diabetes? What are the processes that turn him from a possible diabetic into a real diabetic? And once you know that, can you reverse or prevent the processes from occurring? Heavy questions, indeed. And today, scientists have begun to find some answers to them, even though they're very far from all the answers.

Dr. Abner Notkins, chief of the Laboratory of Oral Medicine at the National Institute of Dental Research, is one of the researchers who has played a massive role in finding these answers. Dr. Notkins has the wonderful ability to simplify some of the most abstract concepts science has ever dealt with.

Wouldn't it be terrific, he asks, if when a child is born, some sort of simple test could be taken that would tell his doctors and family what diseases he'd be likely to come down with during his lifetime? You could kind of "stamp a code on his bottom" as soon as he was born, and the family and doctors would know to what diseases he was genetically susceptible; and maybe they could even, if medical science allowed it by then, do something to preclude his getting that disease.

Well, genetic markers work in somewhat that fashion. Just as each person has a blood group he/she belongs to (Type A blood, Type B blood, etc.), each person also belongs to gene groups. Certain genes produce substances called HLA antigens, which are proteins on the surfaces of many body cells, including the beta cells in the pancreas that produce insulin. HLA antigens have a job: they are part of the body's immune system for spotting and wiping out intruders like bacteria or viruses. Now, there are various kinds of HLA antigens; but scientists have discovered that people with certain HLA antigens, and especially the antigens DR3 and DR4, seem to be more susceptible to insulin-dependent diabetes. Researchers have found out, as a matter of fact, that 90 percent of all children with diabetes have DR3 or DR4.

But, Dr. Notkins cautions, what this means is, "If you're of that particular HLA type, the likelihood of coming down with diabetes is greater than if you're not of that type. That's all it says. It doesn't mean that a child born with DR3 of DR4 *will* come down with diabetes because many people in the population who are DR3 or DR4 do not get diabetes.

"These markers are like a broad paint stripe saying that certain individuals are at a little bit higher risk of developing a disease. Now we're trying to develop this further and get other genetic markers, which will pin down a little more closely those individuals who are at highest risk. There have been studies in families done which indicate that if one child has diabetes and the second child has the same HLA structure, the likelihood of the second child coming down with diabetes is increased maybe fifty-fold over what it would be otherwise . . . and we're looking for more markers to hone it down even further. And we're finding them.

"We've discovered, for example, that many, many children with juvenile diabetes also have auto-antibodies (antibodies that react with their own pancreas tissues) in their bodies . . . and they have these auto-antibodies before they come down with the disease. So that's another prognostic indicator. If you can show that genetic markers *or* auto-antibodies help you predict who's going to come down with the disease, you might be able to do so before they get the disease or at an early stage of that disease. If it turns out to be an immunological process, you might be able to treat these immunological abnormalities and either prevent or retard the disease."

That, then, is the value of genetic markers and one of the important goals of today's researchers. If doctors can learn to tell which people are genetically susceptible to insulin-dependent diabetes, and if diabetes is ultimately found to arise from a virus or other invader, then, theoretically, scientists will be able to watch carefully those youngsters who are most genetically prone to the disease and to find a vaccine that can immunize them against ever getting diabetes, despite the genetic propensities. Which brings us to the next great research drive . . .

Vaccines

Vaccines are modified viruses which, when injected, protect people against getting certain diseases. There has been evidence that some cases of insulin-dependent diabetes are triggered by viral infection—and viral infections are among those that respond to vaccines. If viruses are eventually implicated in more than just a few cases of diabetes, and if the virus or viruses can be identified, then it may be possible to develop a vaccine that will, at long last, be a preventative. Preventing insulin-dependent diabetes will put the Juvenile Diabetes Foundation joyfully and thankfully out of business. How far along are we toward realizing that goal?

Dr. Abner Notkins and his research team at the National Institutes of Health have made recent long strides in this direction that are exciting the entire community of people profoundly involved in diabetes research. The team has found that in experimental animals, like mice, there are viruses that produce a diabetes that is very similar to insulin-dependent diabetes in humans. In certain of the mice are genetic markers that point to their susceptibility to the disease, and these mice, when exposed to the particular diabetes-causing virus EMC (encephalomyocarditis), come down with diabetes. Other mice, without the foretelling genetic markers, do not come down with diabetes even when exposed to the same virus.

Over the last few months, Dr. Notkins and his team have developed a vaccine to immunize the mice that have been infected with EMC. And this vaccine, marvel of marvels, has prevented the development of viral-induced diabetes in 100 percent of the mice.

Now this, as Dr. Notkins says, is wonderful news for mice; but what does it mean for humans?

Well, it means that *if* viruses do turn out to be a major cause of diabetes in humans, you might be able to prevent diabetes with a vaccine.

"The nice part is that we do have now a virus in mice," says Dr. Notkins, "that can produce the acute metabolic changes and long-term complications of diabetes, and now, we can completely prevent diabetes by giving a vaccine to mice. An animal model is complete. *If* we find that viruses are a major cause of diabetes in humans, I would think that the possibilities of developing a vaccine for it would be very high."

And science has gone one step further. The research team found that a person's immune response may also turn against and destroy the insulin-producing beta cells of the pancreas. But the group has been able to suppress the immune system from making these "auto-antibodies" in laboratory animals, and therefore has prevented the development of diabetes caused by auto-immunity in these laboratory animals.

Where does this leave us? When scientists find out whether their vaccines for viruses and immune responses have meaning and application in humans, the next step is a preventative (like the Salk vaccine for polio) to be given as a routine matter to protect children against insulin-dependent diabetes. What a day that will be—if it comes!

New Insulin Delivery Systems

One of the problems of the insulin infusion pump is that it delivers insulin according to the programming of the patient; as devised and used at present, it does not have automatic sensors to tell it how to deliver insulin precisely when or in the amounts that the body's functioning needs require.

Professor Anthony Cerami and Assistant Professor Michael Brownlee are working on such a reliable glucose delivery system. They recently told listeners in a seminar sponsored by JDF that a plant protein called lectin "reversibly binds" to sugars. That means that if sugar molecules are attached to insulin, the insulin can then be temporarily joined with lectin. As glucose levels rise, the glucose replaces the modified insulin, releasing it into the patient's blood. Now, the problem is to develop a safe and reliable delivery system. One possibility would be an implantable hollow-fiber device containing the soluble lectin-sugar-insulin combination. The device, when perfected, will retain the lectin but permit glucose to enter and the insulin to pass to the blood. Because glucose levels could be controlled more narrowly in this "time capsule" device, many of the diabetic complications could probably be forestalled.

At Last ... The Study That Should Find the Answer to the Question

In late 1982, Dr. Lester Salans, director of the National Institute of Arthritis, Diabetes and Digestive and Kidney Diseases, announced an unprecedentedly complete nationwide clinical trial that will involve twenty-one prestigious medical centers. The aim of the study is to find out, once and for all, whether tight control of blood glucose levels prevents, delays, or lessens the development of early complications that affect the blood vessels. If the answer is found to be Yes, then the question that's been on the lips of every diabetic will finally have real meaning: Does it really help when I keep my blood sugar tightly controlled?

Dr. Salans says, "Never before has such a large-scale study of the most controversial issue in diabetes been undertaken. Although most doctors have a feeling that high blood sugar and complications are related, there has been no quantitative controlled data to affirm their feelings. The study should take ten or eleven years, if all goes well."

The development of the insulin pump and devices for home blood glucose monitoring have made it feasible to conduct such a study. If the answer to the question turns out to be a resounding Yes—as many of us at JDF believe it will be—then using methods of tighter control will cut down on the complications of eye, heart, kidney, and neurological disease so common to insulin-dependent diabetes.

6 THE STORY OF JDF

A WISH, A DREAM, AN ANGER—THE STORY OF JDF

The other day, I was slamming balls around with Cheryl Tiegs and Dina Merrill. I, in my tennis whites, looking sweaty and less than glamorous next to those shining stars, missing more points than I made, was still uncontrollably happy. How come happy? Because the occasion was the annual Juvenile Diabetes Foundation tennis tournament, and JDF, the baby I'd birthed in pain, seen through a precarious and iffy infancy and a struggling, strength-gathering childhood, was finally coming of solid age. JDF, which started out because I could think of no other way to find answers for my child Larry, was now finding answers for millions of other insulin-dependent diabetics around the world.

I look at Larry today, that kid of mine, and he's married to wonderful Amy, and he's tanned and strong and productive and optimistic—*and he has a future*. Although there's no cure for him yet, there's infinitely more possibility than there was fifteen years ago because of the efforts of the thousands who have come to be part of the painfully birthed JDF. It's no wonder I felt terrific at the tennis tournament.

I didn't always feel so terrific.

In 1968, for instance, I cried a lot. The tears were always there, right behind my eyes. The pain sat, lumpish, in a stone in my chest. I'd read and read about the thing that had hit our family, the diabetes thing; I'd read about shortened life expectancy, blindness, kidney problems, and every time I looked at my son's sturdy, passionate-with-life little body, I felt weak with fear. There was no way out because I couldn't buy all the Pollyanna hope that friends and doctors had been trying to sell. I read the books, you see. Even though I didn't understand it all, I understood enough.

One day, Dr. Robert Kaye, Larry's personal physician and a giant in the field of diabetes, pronounced Larry "fine as usual" after his three-month check-up and I couldn't stand it.

"But he's NOT fine!" I exploded. "He has insulin reactions, he'll never be like other children, and he has God knows what in front of him. So, he's not fine at all. Admit it. And there's nothing I can do but sit by and watch him be sick for all of his life."

Kaye turned to me, looked at me hard, and said something he'd never said before.

"I think if we had enough money, Lee, we could cure diabetes."

There it was. The words were out. There *was* something to be done. I was naive, I was terrified for my son who was suffering so needlessly, and I thought for a second about the millions of other children in the same boat. And I made a rash promise.

"If it's money you need," I said, "we'll get it."

Sure we'll get it. I was a woman who didn't know the price of a dozen eggs, let alone a test tube or a microscope. Not to mention the price of a scientist who could be convinced to spend his entire life trying to find a cure for my kid. What did I know about grass roots movements? What did I know about asking for government handouts? At home, my husband paid the phone bill, which seemed pretty complicated to my eyes. Things did not look promising for my promise. But *still,* Bob Kaye had put it so simply: money equals cure. There was no choice.

Dr. Kaye gave me a list of his patients and I stared at it blankly. What could I say to these people without seeming to intrude into lives that involved suffering quietly and coping as best as possible with their own fears. How would *I* feel if a stranger, out of the blue, called me and asked me to give time, money, and, maybe worst of all, the truth about my own feelings of guilt and inadequacy in dealing with my son's disease? I had an idea how I might feel because a few years ago, I'd had a shot at trying to share the horror. The shot went blindly off.

Soon after Larry was diagnosed, I'd managed to find two women whose children also had the disease. Oh, I had a million questions for them. Could you ever really go on vacation again? Was there a place to buy quality syringes? Should I tell Larry's friends about his disease? Even more painful were the personal questions that were consuming me. I felt monstrously guilty, for one thing. Could I have somehow prevented this disease if I'd been more observant, more careful? Was it my fault? Was it Edwin's fault? Did anyone else have arguments with their spouses about the way to handle things?

I called the first mother. Cool, cool, polite. Distant. She made light of her child's diabetes. She didn't want to talk. She sure didn't want to cry and share and maybe even wring her hands with me. She obliquely suggested I try to be more mature about the whole thing.

I called the second mother. She denied that her son had diabetes. She hung up.

I was more alone than ever. They wanted private sorrow. I wanted catharsis.

Somehow, I did manage to find three other women. Nessa Stern, just moved to Philadelphia from Los Angeles; Rickey Wagman, the sister of TV producer Chuck Barris; and Connie Lakow. All had diabetic children, and together we formed the most elemental of women's self-help groups. We came before women's liberation and we didn't know about sisterhood and power. All we knew was that we needed the long telephone conversations in which we released our tensions and frustrations. We needed to cry, dissect our mistakes, talk about how *angry* we were with, sometimes, even the kid who was ill for getting us into all this. How angry we were with cavalier doctors, spouses who didn't share the burdens, ourselves for not being able to take away the hurts. And in our togetherness, somehow we found strength to get so angry at the disease we wanted to KILL it.

That's the thought that spurred me on the day I got Bob Kaye's patient list. I wanted to KILL that disease. Even though I knew enlisting allies in a fight that made other people uncomfortable would not be easy, it was a matter of life and death for me to do it . . . as much for my own psyche as for Larry's health, I think. And of course, I'd promised the doctor I'd do it. It was time to start.

May 7, 1970   Eighty people invited to a cocktail party at my home. Eighty rich people, poor people, Jewish, Christian, atheist people; eighty strangers, eighty parents who recognized each other from the pain in the eyes. Eighty parents of kids who had juvenile diabetes. We just may do it, I thought. These people may just pull it together. The code of silence was broken by desperation.

Bob Kaye spoke to us about his hope that if we made some money and some noise, we just might catalyze the medical community to action. No one had ever before attempted such a grass roots organization for diabetes research, he cautioned us. We were beyond caution. We had nothing to lose.

The following week I handed in my resignation as a programmer at a local public television station, put my career plans on hold, and with Connie and Nessa and a promise from eighty volunteers, began laying the groundwork for a volunteer health organization that three months later would be officially chartered and born as the Juvenile Diabetes Foundation.

And what a beginning that was! We depended, as Tennessee Williams would have it, on the kindness of strangers but also on the kindness of relatives. My own relative, my husband, happened to own a suburban apartment building which had a single room so cramped and uncomfortable he hadn't been able to find a paying tenant. We grabbed it! We also grabbed whatever stuff we could cadge from his supply closet: a broken-down copy machine on its way to the dump, somebody's throw-away typewriter, rolls of stamps, blunted pencils, worn office furniture. A public relations agency headed by the father of a diabetic child drew up a logo and brochure free. The law firm of Gold, Bowman & Korman drew up a charter and set aside its fee. And the mothers, awakened to the possibilities of hope for their children, began to arrive at our makeshift office to type, telephone, and talk when their children were at school.

We offered family memberships for $5.00 each, sold cake and cookies on street corners (hoping no diabetics were buying), and once built an entire luncheon around a hurried ten-minute appearance by Muriel Humphrey, who happened to be stumping through town with her husband, Hubert. We grabbed at every excuse, every ploy to raise money. We were shameless. We wrote personal notes to our friends and relatives explaining what it was like to be the mother of a juvenile diabetic, telling them what we hoped to win for our children through JDF, and asking for their big bucks. Big bucks didn't flow, I'm sure I don't have to tell you.

But then the magic happened, the miracles began. We'd be down to our last dollar and talking about failure when a check for $100 to pay the heat bill would materialize from someone, unsolicited. Tennis pro Billy Talbert, an insulin-dependent diabetic, called and asked if we'd be interested in a few truckloads of tomatoes a farmer friend of his had offered to donate. Would we! We had the tomatoes auctioned off at a New York City produce market and the sale brought several thousand dollars—saving us, once again, from financial collapse.

We wheeled and dealed, pleaded and reasoned, and at the end of our first year we gave Bob Kaye $10,000 for research at Children's Hospital. It felt like a million to us. It was our down payment on a cure.

But it was a drop in the vast bucket of what had to be done. We came to the conclusion that we could sell cookies until cancer and the common cold were cured and we still wouldn't raise enough money to make a serious difference to our children. We had to grow up, go where the big guys went. We had to go to the U.S. government, which at the time was allotting a pittance of $6 million a year (smaller than any other disease appropriation administered by the National Institutes of Health) to diabetes.

We had a terrific argument. Just think what the government could save if a cure for diabetes was found. Why, every year they gave billions from social agencies to diabetics who could no longer take care of themselves. I was determined to catch someone's ear who would hear me out.

Early Morning, 1971　The scene is a Metroliner to Washington, DC. Speeding along are Dr. Lester Baker of Children's Hospital in Philadelphia, my husband, and I. We're on our way to meet Senator Richard S. Schweiker, a Pennsylvania Republican who had agreed to hear our appeal for legislation to spur diabetes research.

Schweiker was to give us five minutes.

Five minutes!

Five minutes to get funding and a future for JDF.

Five minutes to lay out a plan, an argument, a good reason why the big guys should help us.

Five minutes to get my son Larry a cure.

I talked fast.

At precisely the end of my five minutes, Senator Schweiker stood up, said goodbye, and disappeared. I was sure we'd failed . . . that I'd wasted those precious minutes.

But we didn't fail . . . we *won!* Schweiker became our very good friend, and his efforts finally led to the creation of a fifteen-member task force to develop a long-range plan to combat diabetes and to establish research, treatment, and education centers throughout the country.

On August 4, 1972, Congress brought about the biggest miracle of all: the enactment of the National Diabetes Mellitus Research and Education Act. By a heartstopping (my heart) coincidence, it happened to be Larry's seventeenth birthday. It was enough to make you cry.

Since then the federal government has appropriated almost $500 *million* to the cause. We're on our way. Dr. Leo Krall of Boston's Joslin Clinic says he now tells his young patients, "Look, you guys, take good care of yourselves. We've got something coming."

What's coming is surely a cure. Not yet, not this year or probably next year, but soon. We know it. And what's more, in the meantime, scientists are now researching ways of stopping the devastating complications of diabetes.

As of this writing, the Juvenile Diabetes Foundation has grown from the crowded little room in Philadelphia to an international network of more than 150 chapters across the United States, Israel, Canada, Brazil, and Italy, and we're still growing in other countries of the world. Of all the diabetes organizations in existence today, we're the largest. Our foremost thrust is still to raise money to be spent in research. Our fondest hope is that the research will, one day, put us out of business. Perhaps the most immediate thing we do best is that person-to-person contact that encourages the parent of a newly diagnosed diabetic to call and say, "Please, please can you help me—I'm scared." And we can help, in more ways than you can imagine. After all, we've been there.

It is my firmly held belief that we have grown so large and have been able to do so much because of our unique philosophy. And it is this: it is the parents, the lay people, the grass roots individuals who needed us and helped us to grow from the start who are the "big bosses" of our organization. Whereas other large organizations tend to leave the running of their vast machinery to the pros, the "experts," we have insisted on the parents—us—being the experts. We've learned that we have the most at stake—and that is our families. We've learned that we are the best advocates for ourselves and that we, yes indeed, we, often uneducated, often scared, often feeling helpless, know more than any scientists or Presidents alive about living with juvenile diabetes. And therefore, *we* intend to have the final say as to where the money goes.

We have on our boards the most distinguished doctors and scientists to be found. We have pursued the finest in their fields and they have consented to participate. But behind every "professional" decision is the Lay Review Board, made up of parents who give approval to every JDF grant; and those grants have come to over $15 million that has flowed from JDF's treasury into laboratories all over the world.

To many, in the beginning, and even now, the set-up seems presumptuous. After all, how can lay people, often equipped only with high school diplomas (and sometimes none at all), be watchdogs over the professionals? The answer is: Carefully. And thoroughly. And absolutely. If we're going to work our butts off to raise money, we want to have a say where it goes. And while our children are waiting for a cure to be found, we don't want one penny of that money siphoned off into unnecessary duplication, graft, unnecessary overhead, bricks and mortar. We have found that there are no mysteries. A complex organization can be run as smoothly and efficiently as a kitchen budget, despite the fact that the "experts" say you need "experts." Which is why you won't find glossy, meaningless brochures, figurehead leaders, or more than a handful of paid employees in our hundreds of volunteer offices. We have succeeded because, as the Bell Telephone people say, we've learned how to reach out and touch people.

This chapter is about wishes and dreams, but it's also about anger. More than fifteen years have passed since Larry was diagnosed as having diabetes. Looking back on those days immediately following the diagnosis, I feel a rising sense of anger. And I feel it every time I think about it. The anger is not directed against the individual doctors who treated him and stabilized his condition—I was lucky to live in a big city and to have had resources on which to draw—but anger at the whole medical community in general. How dared they say, as they did, to many of us, "If your child takes his insulin, exercises regularly, and watches his diet, he'll be just fine"? How dared they not have told us of the crippling devastation diabetes could wreak—*even if you were good and did all the good things?* Didn't they know? Sure, they did. How dared they say that diabetes was an "okay" disease and we should be grateful it wasn't something much more serious.

I don't think it was our fault that we swallowed those lines—hook, line, and sinker. That we lived with the soothing balm, the Big Lie, until, for many of us, the time bombs exploded. But still, how did it happen that an entire population of diabetics and their families bought propaganda that made it easy for the doctors to "handle" the emotions of families? I often wonder how those doctors, who knew better, slept soundly at night after telling parents about the "okay" disease.

According to the National Diabetes Data Group of the National Institutes of Health, there are certain undeniable facts.

FACT: One in every twenty persons in the United States is now affected by diabetes—over 11 million people.

FACT: In the past six years alone, over 3.6 million new cases of diabetes have been diagnosed, about 10 percent of them children. There's been a *sixfold increase* in prevalence since the mid-1930s.

FACT: Diabetes causes almost 50 percent of amputations of the foot and leg among adults.

FACT: Diabetes causes 20 percent of all cases of kidney failure, and 15 percent of all blindness.

FACT: Diabetes in pregnant women causes about 1300 fetal and infant deaths; gestational diabetes contributes an additional 900 fetal deaths.

FACT: Twenty-five percent of diabetics have heart disease, and diabetes is one of the four major risk factors for cardiovascular diseases.

FACT: Diabetics have twice as much disability as non-diabetics, and spend twice as many days in the hospital as persons without this disorder.

FACT: More than a quarter of all diabetics require hospitalization each year; 34,000 deaths in the Unites States are directly attributable to diabetes, and an additional 100,000 deaths to its complications.

FACT: The United States ranks among the five nations in the world with the highest rate of mortality due to diabetes.

It's not an okay disease!

I think the medical community had a responsibility to tell us the truth, and it was a certain kind of arrogance and non-caring that led them to lull us into complacency. And I think that if the word was out that insulin did not cure diabetes; that exercise and diet were important, sure, but that cure was the thing to shoot for—then an organization like JDF would have been founded long ago, by a man or a woman like me who couldn't bear to be soothed and lulled by lies one minute longer.

JDF went into business to go out of business. It's a singleminded group with one aim: to find a cure and to disband. Heretical as it sounds, I and many other parents feel that other organizations which are doctor groups before they are patient-parent support groups are not always interested in going out of business.

So there we are. As long as we have fight in us, we'll not bow to special interest groups. We'll not take commands, but we'll educate ourselves and be our own best self-advocates. As long as we have fight in us—and what parent doesn't have enough to last a lifetime?—our kids have a much better chance of

- *Not* going blind
- *Not* dying early
- *Not* having limbs amputated
- *Not* giving up lives of promise, family, and love.

We're not there yet, but we know the truths. And the truths will set us . . . you know what.

Years ago, a letter came to me from a woman in India whose 6-year-old daughter was awaiting death, so sick from diabetes was she. Although JDF had never before attempted quite such a dramatic rescue, we raced around buying airplane tickets, and flew the parents and daughter to Children's Hospital in Philadelphia. There, under the care of Dr. Lester Baker, the child was properly stabilized and sent home with a supply of insulin, syringes, information, and a future.

Her mother wrote me, recently, because we have stayed in touch.

"I see the day when our children will throw their syringes into the sea," she said. "And we will celebrate."

I already celebrate. I celebrate the thousands of people who have helped me keep the promise I made to Dr. Kaye when I was young and green. I celebrate the struggle and the agonies and the victories of the insulin-dependent diabetics, who are, I don't know why, the nicest, smartest, funniest, most special people in the world. I celebrate the daily, ongoing search of the *dedicated* doctors and scientists who have made life worth living again, for so many of us.

I celebrate the beauty and the growth of the Juvenile Diabetes Foundation—the grass roots baby support system of knowledge and hope.

EPILOGUE

And What Happened to the Nine-Year-Old Kid, Larry Ducat?
Does He Live Happily Ever After?

This book started out with my son. It's fitting that the book should end with a portrait of what he's become and what he hopes to be.

But let my co-author, Sherry, do it. My eyes mist too much when I look hard at him:

For months now, I'd been hearing about the nine-year-old for whom a multi-million-dollar research organization was invented, and even though I knew better, I half expected it would be that same little boy who would be showing up for dinner. Who did show up could have won the Mr. Health contest. He radiated health, strength, intelligence; sandy-haired, with strong, classic features, Larry Ducat is one of the new breed of self-assured young men who look directly into your eyes as you speak. Gently but gravely, he muses about his past and his present.

When he was small, he remembers seeing hordes of people, shepherded by his mother, bustling around to raise money for diabetes.

"My mother was this lady," he says, "who everybody told me put diabetes research on the map. I felt protected. We had access to the best doctors, the newest research, the most optimistic thinking. I didn't really see diabetes as much of a problem."

Oh, sure, he thought about complications. He'd play his guitar for hours with his eyes closed just to see how it would feel to go blind. But he never really thought it would happen. He went surfing and he ran track and, in deference to the disease, he'd run an extra five miles before he drank his share of a keg of beer. He was seventeen, then eighteen, then nineteen, and there were always those promises the researchers were making—"in the next five years, there'll be a cure"—and then, after five years, "in the next five years, there'll *surely* be a cure."

He took his shots and he learned the latest news about diabetes, and he grew up. Amy came into his life and they fell in love. They both weren't too worried about the disease; they hardly even discussed it except to talk about what if they were to have children *if* they decided to get married. Who was worried was Amy's parents. They thought about diabetes a lot. "Date him, but don't marry him," they advised. "He's bound to have complications; he may even die early, leaving you with little ones, alone."

"I couldn't reassure them," says Amy. "But I'm stubborn. We loved each other and just didn't see diabetes as a negative force that could keep us apart."

They were married. Amy was twenty: a clear-eyed, ingenuous, radiant bride. Larry was twenty-five, the strong-jawed groom on top of the wedding cake. Fairy tale come true.

And it still is. At dinner with me, they touch each other as much as possible and they laugh at their private jokes. They're delicious, this young couple, and you want to hug them.

But it's not all Hans Christian Andersen. For one thing, Larry got quite sick last month: he threw up horribly because of a stomach virus and he had a powerful insulin reaction.

"He didn't know who I was," says Amy. "He didn't recognize me. I was so scared. *He didn't know me!*"

For another thing, Larry recently found out from his ophthalmologist that he has the beginnings of some eye complications. Those are the realities. They're starting. They may not go much further . . . but they may. And they cannot be ignored.

"Of all my life, this is probably the toughest time for me," says Larry. "For the first time, I know I'm vulnerable. I used to live in the closet, as most diabetics do, with this disease. Pretending I was normal, not talking about it, denying it. All of a sudden, it's pretty scary to hear about this eye thing. It's depressing."

So he rushes to get it all in. One of the things that often happens to diabetics, says Larry, is that, "If you have the feeling that your time on this planet is cut short even by a split minute, it has a ripple effect on all your life decisions." So you want to do everything fast. You hurry up, afraid you might have to miss out on it. Larry Ducat left architecture school a year and a half early because he wanted to get out in the world and get started on his fortune. For the same reason, he wants to start a family soon. But Amy isn't so sure.

"Look, I'm very young, I have my career to think about, and, and . . ." (and you just know this is the real *and*) "I'm not so sure I could handle having a child who is diabetic, if that should happen, even though I know the odds are pretty much in our favor against having a child with the disease."

They're pretty candid, these two. If anyone makes it, you figure they should. "We really do want to plan for the future," says Larry; "but it's hard when you don't know how long or how solid a future you'll have."

"And maybe my mother was right," says Amy. "Maybe I'll be left with nine kids and no money. And Kasha the cat who has acne. We have to live pretty much for now—that's the only real frame of reality we have. So if Larry is cranky because his blood sugar is low, I try to understand and stuff him with sugar. I DO get mad when he doesn't talk to me when he feels sick—that gets me maddest."

"I *can't* talk to you because I'm non-verbal then. I don't even know I'm getting sick, half the time," Larry interjects. "You know what's particularly aggravating for *me*? That we can never take a rest or vacation from diabetes. I hate the sound of the very word. It's the ugliest-sounding word I ever heard in my whole life. For years, I said diabet-ess instead of diabet-ees because I hoped it sounded better, but it doesn't. Still, I'm used to it now, and I think I'd rather have it than any other awful illness. I work with my father in the hospital-building business, and I see a lot of terrible diseases. I'd rather be a healthy diabetic than a sissy asthmatic, say, even if that brings the wrath of the asthmatics of the world down on me.

"What's our best hope? A cure. Every diabetic thinks about a cure at least ten times a day. Actually, if you're a guy, you think about sex every thirty seconds, and getting rid of this monkey on your back every forty seconds. Through my mother's efforts, I've always had a real sense of hope that diabetes would be cured in my active lifetime—before complications of a serious nature occur. I still have that hope; but sometimes I tend to question the time clocks of the scientists. Another five years? Another? I get tired of hearing that."

So they grapple daily with decisions and adjustments, this young couple you want to hug. And they're realistic. A few years ago, Larry helped to choose the theme for JDF from a John Ciardi poem. "Whatever magic you expect from dreams is heavy on the air," reads the message. Larry Ducat has dreams that are magnificent, but he wouldn't swear to magic. Larry and Amy have a warm and nurturing love, but they don't buy false promises of forever. They wouldn't swear to forever, at all. They only know that they love each other, and they're taking care of Larry's disease as well as possible, with Larry testing his blood up to six times a day. They even have their friends testing their own blood, squeamishly, sometimes green of complexion, but happy to share the burden in even the smallest ways. The young

Ducats, you could say, are playing it by ear.

And one more thing. Lee can't say it but I can without fear that I'll be thought unobjective.

Larry Ducat is a doll. He's *worth* founding a multi-million-dollar organization for. He's worth a lot more. He's worth a cure.

RESOURCES:
WHERE TO GO...

Throughout this book, we've stressed the absolute necessity of *self-advocacy,* which simply means making sure you or your family gets the very best available in treatment. It can make all the difference in the world to health and long life when you're dealing with the intricacies of diabetes.

But where to find the best? What follows are comprehensive lists of specialists in insulin-dependent diabetes. You probably cannot find another more complete list specifically geared to the disease.

There is an enormous range in the quality of care available to diabetes patients in this country. Fortunately, although there are medical practitioners who are careless and ill informed, there are also splendid doctors who are concerned, compassionate, and gifted in their insistence on the best and most up-to-date medical care available. And there are extraordinary centers and hospitals that offer care, advice, and treatment for the patient with diabetes. While of course not every excellent doctor and hospital is named here (your own may be among those not listed), we offer enough of a demographic spread of reputable medical sources to give you choices.

In the end, the more you listen and learn from the experts, the more of an expert you will become, and that is the secret of the best self-care. There's no magic and no myth to diabetes treatment; the finest doctors in the world will tell you that. Informed decisions about your own treatment, based on education, common sense, and recent medical advances rather than blind faith, are the way to go. Whether you live in the proverbial little mining town or a big city, whether you're rich or poor—you ought to seek out and insist on the best. You deserve it.

I. THE DOCTORS AND THE HOSPITALS

Listed below are some pediatricians, all of them members of the Lawson Wilkins Pediatric Endocrine Society, who are, in our judgment, expert in the treatment of children who have diabetes.

A. Pediatricians

Lester Baker, M.D.
Children's Hospital of Philadelphia
34th & Civic Center Boulevard
Philadelphia, PA 19104
(215) 387-6165

Dennis Bier, M.D.
Metabolism Division
Washington University School of
    Medicine
St. Louis, MO 63110
(314) 454-2935

David M. Brown, M.D.
Department of Pediatrics
University of Minnesota Hospitals
Minneapolis, MN 55455
(612) 544-7932

Ian M. Burr, M.D.
Department of Pediatrics
School of Medicine
Vanderbilt University
Nashville, TN 37203
(615) 322-7427

Eleanor Colle, M.D.
Montreal Children's Hospital
Montreal, Quebec, Canada
(514) 937-8511 ext. 346

Marvin Cornblath, M.D., Special
    Assistant to the Scientific
    Director
National Institutes of Health (NICHD)
Clinical Center 13N260
Bethesda, MD 20014
(301) 496-6683

Henry Dolger, M.D.
11 East 86th Street
New York, NY 10028

Allan L. Drash, M.D.
The Children's Hospital
125 DeSoto Street
Pittsburgh, PA 15213
(412) 681-7700 ext. 431

Donnell Etzwiler, M.D.
St. Louis Park Medical Center
5000 West 39th Street
Minneapolis, MN 55416
(612) 920-6742

Kenneth H. Gabbay, M.D.
Children's Hospital Medical Center
Research Building G628
300 Longwood Avenue
Boston, MA 02115
(617) 734-6000 ext. 3943

Fredda Ginsberg-Fellner, M.D.
Department of Pediatrics (Annenberg
    17-24)
Mount Sinai School of Medicine
11 East 100th Street
New York, NY 10029
(212) 650-6936

Richard A. Guthrie, M.D.
Department of Pediatrics
Wichita State University
University of Kansas School of
    Medicine
2221 North Hillside
Wichita, KS 67219
(316) 689-3097

Robert L. Jackson, M.D.
Department of Pediatrics M-769
University of Missouri Medical Center
Columbia, MO 65201
(314) 882-6979

Robert Kaye, M.D.
Hahnemann Medical College and
    Hospital
Department of Pediatrics
230 North Broad Street
Philadelphia, PA 19102
(215) 448-7767

Noel K. Maclaren, M.D.
Department of Pediatrics
University of Florida College of
    Medicine
Gainesville, FL 32610
(904) 392-4495

Maria New, M.D.
Department of Pediatrics
The New York Hospital
Cornell Medical Center
525 East 68th Street
New York, NY 10021
(212) 472-5658

Elsa P. Paulsen, M.D.
Department of Pediatrics
University of Virginia School of
  Medicine
Charlottesville, VA 22901
(804) 924-5065

Arlan L. Rosenbloom
Department of Pediatrics
Box J-296
University of Florida College of
  Medicine
Gainesville, FL 32610
(904) 392-3331

Julio Santiago, M.D.
Department of Pediatrics
Washington University School of
  Medicine
500 South Kingshighway
St. Louis, MO 63178
(314) 454-6046

Mark A. Sperling, M.D.
Department of Pediatric Endocrinology
Children's Hospital Medical Center
Elland & Bethesda Avenues
Cincinnati, OH 45229
(513) 559-4200

Luther B. Travis, M.D.
Department of Pediatrics
University of Texas Medical Branch
Galveston, TX 77550
(713) 765-2538

B. Physician Specialists for Young Adults

Dr. Robert Bradley
Joslin Clinic
1 Joslin Place
Boston, MA 02215

Dr. Harvey C. Knowles, Jr.
University of Cincinnati College of
  Medicine
231 Bethesda Avenue
Cincinnati, OH 45267

Dr. Arthur Rubenstein
University of Chicago Hospitals &
  Clinics
950 East 59th Street
Chicago, IL 60637

Dr. Charles R. Shuman
Temple University Hospital
3401 North Broad Street
Philadelphia, PA 19140

Dr. Fred W. Whitehouse
2799 West Grand Boulevard
Detroit, MI 48238

C. Physician Specialists for Eye Problems

If you have concerns about retinopathy, the following are some of the finest clinical research centers that specialize in eye problems stemming from diabetes. The doctors listed for each center are the principal investigators for that center's participation in the ongoing Diabetic Retinopathy Study. Any one of them can be relied on to treat you expertly or to help you find a specialist in your own area.

Albany Medical College
Albany, NY
 Stephen Feman, M.D.
 W. A. J. van Heuven, M.D.
 Aaron Kassoff, M.D.

Johns Hopkins Hospital
Wilmer Institute
Baltimore, MD
 Stuart Fine, M.D.
 Arnall Patz, M.D.
 Thaddeus Prout, M.D.

Joslin Clinic
Boston, MA
 Lloyd Aiello, M.D.
 Robert Bradley, M.D.

Massachusetts Eye and Ear Infirmary
Boston, MA
 Evangelos Gragoudas, M.D.
 Donald Martin, M.D.
 J. Wallace McMeel, M.D.

UCLA Center for Health Sciences
Jules Stein Eye Institute
Los Angeles, CA
 Stanley Kopelow, M.D.
 Bradley Straatsma, M.D.

University of Illinois
Chicago, IL
 Morton Goldberg, M.D.
 Felipe Huamonte, M.D.
 Gholam Peyman, M.D.

University of Iowa
Iowa City, IA
 John Mensher, M.D.
 Robert Watzke, M.D.

University of Miami
Bascom Palmer Eye Institute
 George Blankenship, M.D.
 Edward Norton, M.D.

University of Minnesota
Minneapolis, MN
 Frederick Goetz, M.D.
 John Harris, M.D.
 William Knobloch, M.D.

University of Puerto Rico
San Juan, PR
 Jose Berrocal, M.D.
 Antonio Ramos, M.D.

University of Utah
Salt Lake City, UT
 William Bohart, M.D.
 Mary Dahl, M.D.
 F. Tempel Riekhf, M.D.

University of Washington
Seattle, WA
 Steven Guzak, M.D.
 Edward McLean, M.D.

University of Wisconsin
Madison, WI
 George Bresnick, M.D.
 Frank Meyers, M.D.
 Guillermo de Venecia, M.D.

Wayne State University
Detroit, MI
 Raymond Margherio, M.D.
 Delbert Nachazel, M.D.

Wills Eye Hospital
Philadelphia, PA
 William Annesley, M.D.
 Brian Leonard, M.D.
 William Tasman, M.D.

Coordinating Center:
University of Maryland
Baltimore, MD
 Argye Hillis, Ph.D.
 Christian Klimt, M.D.
 Genell Knatterud, Ph.D., Principal
 Investigator

Fundus Photograph Reading Center
University of Wisconsin
Madison, WI
 Matthew Davis, M.D., Principal
 Investigator
 Alasdair MacCormick, Ph.D.
 Paul Segal, M.D.

D. Hospital Specialists

The following hospitals are noted for special areas of diabetes care:

Barnes Hospital, St. Louis
The primary teaching hospital for Washington University, this institution has been a pioneer in insulin treatment for juvenile diabetics.

Brigham & Women's Hospital, Boston
A Harvard Medical School affiliate and a top research center, this was the site of the world's first kidney transplant.

Columbia-Presbyterian Medical Center, New York City
As a leading care center for pregnant women and their newborns, this hospital also specializes in treating children with birth defects. It pioneered laser surgery for the eye.

Duke University Medical Center, Durham, N.C.
This is a top treatment center for chronic pain, anorexia nervosa, and diabetes. It is also the site of a $137,000 federal study to determine whether diabetics can use relaxation techniques and other behavioral training to lower blood sugar.

Johns Hopkins Hospital, Baltimore
Johns Hopkins is the home of the renowed Wilmer Eye Institute.

Massachusetts General Hospital, Boston
The largest hospital in New England and the primary teaching center for Harvard Medical School, Mass General boasts an outstanding roster of heart and diabetes specialists.

New York Hospital-Cornell Medical Center, New York City
Known in medical circles for its study of high blood pressure and for the Rogosin Kidney Center, a leading transplant and dialysis facility.

Stanford University Medical Center, Stanford, California
One of the top U.S. cardiology and transplant centers.

University of California at San Francisco Hospitals, San Francisco
A famous West Coast center for treating diabetes.

Yale-New Haven Hospital, New Haven, Connecticut
Home of the clinical center for insulin pump therapy.

II. RESEARCH AND TRAINING CENTERS

Are you interested in the very latest information as to what's going on in the world of research? The following diabetes research and training centers and the doctors listed for each are among the most prestigious in the nation. A call to any one of them will either result in the information you seek or a suggestion as to where to find such information.

Dr. Charles M. Clark, Jr.
Department of Medicine
Indiana University Medical Center
1100 West Michigan Street
Indianapolis, IN 46202
(317) 635-7401 ext. 2266 or 2267
    (VA) 264-3574

Dr. Oscar Crofford
Diabetes Research and Training
    Center
Vanderbilt University School of
    Medicine
Nashville, TN 37232
(615) 322-2197

Dr. William H. Daughaday
Washington University Diabetes
    Research & Training Center
660 South Euclid Avenue
St. Louis, MO 63110
(314) 454-3387

Dr. Stefan Fajans
Endocrinology & Metabolism Division
University of Michigan School of
    Medicine
Ann Arbor, MI 48104
(313) 764-4165 or 763-5256 (admin.)

Dr. James B. Field
Diabetes Research Center
Baylor College of Medicine
1200 Moursund Avenue
Houston, TX 77030
(713) 791-4244

Dr. Normal S. Fleischer
Albert Einstein College of Medicine
1300 Morris Park Avenue
Bronx, NY 10461
(212) 430-2908

Dr. Daryl K. Granner
Department of Internal Medicine
University of Iowa College of Medicine
Iowa City, IA 52242
(319) 338-0581 ext.465

Dr. Joseph Larner
Diabetes Research and Training
    Center
University of Virginia
Charlottesville, VA 22903
(804) 924-5207 or 924-5869 (admin.)

Dr. Franz Matschinsky
Diabetes-Endocrinology Center
University of Pennsylvania School of
    Medicine
Philadelphia, PA 19104
(215) 622-3165

Dr. Daniel Porte, Jr.
Diabetes-Endocrinology Center
University of Washington
1131 14th Avenue South, QR 8
Seattle, WA 98195
(206) 762-1010 ext. 493 or
(FTS) 396-1431, 1493

Dr. Howard Tager
Department of Biochemistry
Cummings Life Science Center
920 East 58th Street
Chicago, IL 60637
(312) 753-3974

III. GENERAL INFORMATION

Do you want the latest statistics on anything having to do with insulin-dependent diabetes? Call or write

The National Diabetes Data Group
   Dr. Maureen Harris
   NIH/NIADDK/DEMD
   Westwood Building, Room 622, Bethesda, MD 20205
   (301) 496-7595

Do you want to be pointed in the right direction for the answers to any questions about insulin-dependent diabetes? Call or write

The National Diabetes Information Clearinghouse
   Mrs. Lois Lipsett
   NIH/NIADDK/DEMD
   Westwood Building, Room 603, Bethesda, MD 20205
   (301) 496-7433

The latest on human insulin ...

These are the kinds of human insulin that are presently available in the United Kingdom, Holland, Germany and the United States from Eli Lilly and Company:

United Kingdom
   Regular   U-40   NPH U-40
                         U-80   U-80
                         U-100   U-100

Holland
   Regular   U-40   NPH U-40

Germany
   Regular   U-40   NPH U-40

   Profil I (10:90 mixture   Profil II U-40 (20:80
   regular and NPH)   mixture regular and NPH)

United States
   Regular   U-100   NPH U-100

   Squibb-Novo human insulin is called Novo and is available in Actrapid and Monotard formulations in Denmark, West Germany, United Kingdom and Ireland, Holland, Sweden, and Switzerland.

IV. DIABETES CLINICAL RESEARCH TRIAL CENTERS AND PRINCIPAL INVESTIGATORS

In Chapter 5, we discussed the extraordinary clinical trial study aimed at finding out the true benefits of controlled blood glucose levels. Taking part in this study are some of the most prestigious medical centers specializing in the treatment of insulin-dependent diabetes, and, of course, some of the most renowned doctors in the field. It's a good list for you to study. Should you have a child who has been diagnosed as a juvenile diabetic, or should you be a young adult who has the disease, any one of the doctors listed at any one of these hospitals, or the doctors they will be able to recommend, would give you the finest care available in the country.

Throughout this book, we have stressed the necessity of having a *specialist* treat your child or you in every aspect of diabetes, whether you need a pediatrician, retinopathy expert, neuropathy expert, or an expert in kidney or cardiovascular problems related to diabetes. If you do not know where to find such experts, these participating centers and their principal investigators will steer you to the right place.

Dr. Lester Baker
Joseph Stokes, Jr., Research Institute
    (University of Pennsylvania)
Children's Hospital of Philadelphia
Philadelphia, PA

Dr. Jose J. Barbosa
University of Minnesota School of
    Medicine
Minneapolis, MN

Dr. John Amory Colwell
Medical University of South Carolina
Charleston, SC

Dr. Oscar Crofford, Chairman
Diabetes Research and Training
    Center
Vanderbilt University School of
    Medicine
Nashville, TN

Dr. Allan L. Drash
The Children's Hospital
Pittsburgh, PA

Dr. John Dupre
University of Western Ontario
University Hospital
London, Ontario, Canada

Dr. Donnell D. Etzwiler
St. Louis Park Medical Center
Research Foundation
Minneapolis, MN

Dr. Saul Genuth
Mount Sinai Hospital
Cleveland, OH

Dr. David Goldstein
University of Missouri—Columbia
    School of Medicine
Columbia, MO

Dr. Lois Jovanovic
Cornell University Medical School
New York, NY

Dr. Abbas E. Kitabchi
University of Tennessee Center for the
    Health Sciences
Memphis, TN

Dr. Rodney A. Lorenz
Diabetes Research and Training
    Center
Vanderbilt University School of
    Medicine
Nashville, TN

Dr. David M. Nathan
Massachusetts General Hospital
Boston, MA

Dr. Jerry P. Palmer
Diabetes Research Center
U.S. PHS Hospital Quarters 8
Seattle, WA

Dr. Lawrence I. Rand
Joslin Diabetes Center, Inc.
Joslin Clinic Division
Boston, MA

Dr. Philip Raskin
University of Texas Health Science
    Center
Southwestern Medical School
Dallas, TX

Dr. Julio V. Santiago
Washington University School of
    Medicine
500 South Kingshighway
St. Louis, MO 63178

Dr. Helmut Gunther Schrott
University of Iowa
Iowa City, IA

Dr. F. John Service
Mayo Foundation
Rochester, MN

Dr. William V. Tamborlane, Jr.
Yale University School of Medicine
New Haven, CT

Dr. Fred Waite Whitehouse
Henry Ford Hospital
Detroit, MI

Dr. Bernard Zinman
Toronto General Hospital
Toronto, Ontario, Canada

V. PROFESSIONAL ORGANIZATIONS AND MANUFACTURERS (FOR RECOMMENDATIONS AND INFORMATION)

American Association of Diabetes
    Educators
North Woodbury Road Box 56
Pitman, NJ 08071
(Write for information on diabetes
    education programs in your
    community)
American Association of
    Ophthalmology
1100 17th Street, N.W.
Washington, DC 20036
(202) 833-3447

American College of Obstetricians and
    Gynecologists
1 East Whacker Drive
Chicago, IL 60601
(312) 222-1600

American Dental Association
211 East Chicago Avenue, Suite 1804
Chicago, IL 60611
(312) 440-2500

American Diabetes Association
2 Park Avenue
New York, NY 10016
(212) 683-7444

American Dietetic Association
430 North Michigan Avenue
Chicago, IL 60610
(312) 751-6166

American Medical Association
535 North Dearborn Street
Chicago, Illinois 60610

American Podiatry Association
20 Chevy Chase Circle, N.W.
Washington, DC 20015
(202) 537-4900

Ames Division
Miles Laboratories, Inc.
1127 Myrtle Street
Elkhart, IN 46515

Becton, Dickinson Consumer Products
Division (B-D)
P.O. Box 5000
Rochelle Park, NJ 07662

Bio-Dynamics, Inc. (Division of
Boehringer Mannheim)
9115 Hague Road
Indianapolis, IN 46250

International Diabetes Federation
3-6 Alfred Place
London WCI E7EE England

Joslin Diabetes Foundation
1 Joslin Place
Boston, MA 02155
(617) 732-2400

Juvenile Diabetes Foundation
23 East 26th Street
New York, NY 10010
(212) 889-7575
(Check in your local phone book for
chapter nearest you)

Eli Lilly & Company
307 East McCarty Street
Indianapolis, IN 46285

Medic Alert Foundation
1000 North Palm Street
Turlock, CA 95380
(209) 632-2371

Monoject (Division of Sherwood
Medical)
1831 Olive Street
St. Louis, MO 63103

National Diabetes Information
Clearinghouse:

(i) 7910 Woodmont Avenue Suite 1811
Bethesda, MD 20014
(301) 654-0897

(ii) 805 15th Street, N.W. Suite 500
Washington, DC 20005
(202) 638-7620

National Institutes of Health
U.S. Department of Health and Human
Services
9000 Rockville Pike
Bethesda, MD 20205
(301) 496-4000

National Kidney Foundation
2 Park Avenue
New York, NY 10016
(212) 889-2210

Nordisk
6500 Rock Spring Drive
Bethesda, MD 20817

Paddock Laboratories
2744 Lyndale Avenue S.
Minneapolis, Minnesota 55408
Toll Free No.: 800-328-5113

Pfizer Laboratories Division
235 East 42nd Street
New York, NY 10017

Squibb-Novo Inc.
120 Alexander Street
Princeton, NJ 08540

Sugarfree Center for Diabetes
5623 Matilija Avenue P.O. Box 2166
Van Nuys, CA 91401
(a mail-order service that provides
materials, diabetes books, self-
care products. Write for free
brochure)

The Upjohn Co.
7000 Portage Road
Kalamazoo, MI 49001

U.S. Department of Health and Human
Services
200 Independence Avenue, S.W.
Washington, DC 20201

VI. INSULIN PUMP MANUFACTURERS

The insulin pump is one of the newest and most interesting forms of treatment today. Your doctor may not be aware that there are many kinds of pumps, at many prices, offering different benefits (and sometimes drawbacks). As an informed diabetic patient, you ought to know the various manufacturers of these pumps so that you can compare qualities and prices to best advantage. Call or write the following for information about their pumps.

Auto-Syringe, Inc.
William D. Arthur
Londonderry Turnpike
Hooksett, NH 03104
(603) 669-9805

Becton, Dickinson & Company
Edward R. Duffie, Jr., M.D., Vice
President
Advanced Business Development
Stanley Street
East Rutherford, NJ 07070
(201) 460-2991

Bio-Dynamics Corp.
Charles Suther
9115 Hague Road
Indianapolis, IN 46250
1-800-428-5074

Delta Medical Industries
George Siposs, President
1579 Sunland Lane
Costa Mesa, CA 92626
(714) 549-0504

Harvard Apparatus
Harold Sossen, Director of Research
& Development
22 Pleasant Street
South Natick, MA 01760
(617) 655-7000

Intermedics, Inc.
David C. Howson, Director of
Marketing for Neurological
Products
P.O. Box 617
Freeport, TX 77541
(713) 233-8611 ext. 1764

Eli Lilly & Company
Cornelius Pettinga, Ph.D., Executive
Vice President
307 East McCarty Street
Indianapolis, IN 46285
(317) 261-2000

Medtronic, Inc.
Kent R. Van Kampen, D.V.M.,
Ph.D.
Director, Drug Administration
Devices Systems Processing
6970 Central Avenue, NE
P.O. Box 1453
Minneapolis, MN 55440
(612) 574-4403

Miles Laboratories, Inc.
Lawrence H. Chanoch, New
Business Development
Manager—Diabetes Systems
Ames Division
P.O. Box 70
Elkhart, IN 46515
(219) 264-8645 ext. 7987

Pacesetter Systems, Inc.
12884 Bradley Ave.
Sylmar, CA 91342
(213) 362-6822

Parker Hannifin
Freddi Fredrickson, R.N., Medical
Products Specialist
Biomedical Products Division
17352 Von Karman Avenue
Irvine, CA 92714
(714) 851-3358 ext. 3669

St. Jude Medical, Inc.
  David Thomas, Ph.D., Regulatory
    Affairs
  1 Lillehei Plaza
  St. Paul, MN 55117
  (612) 483-2000

The Infusaid Corp.
  Frank Prosl, Chief Engineer
  1075 Providence Highway
  Sharon, MA 02067
  (617) 668-3050

Travenol Laboratories
  Lu Wolf
  Route 120 & Wilson Road
  Round Lake, IL 60013
  (312) 546-6311 ext. 2077

VII. MENTAL HEALTH

Everyone knows that stress control is an integral part of diabetes management. There are any number of professional individuals and organizations that can help you to achieve tranquility. For recommendations, call or write to:

The National Institute of Mental Health
Public Inquiries Office
5600 Fishers Lane
Rockville, MD 20857
(301) 443-4795

And check into

- *Silva Mind Control*
- *Yoga*
- *Transcendental Meditation*
- *Biofeedback*

These different techniques geared to create relaxation and peacefulness are often listed in the telephone book separately or under *"Psychological Services."*

Individual mental health professionals—psychiatrists, psychologists, and other counselors—are best found through your own doctor or from recommendations of the psychology and psychiatry departments of large teaching hospitals.

VIII. BOOKS WE THINK ARE FINE

Diabetes by Sarah R. Riedman. New York: Franklin Watts, 1980.

An Instructional Aid on Juvenile Diabetes Mellitus by Luther B. Travis, M.D.
  (Obtainable from the American Diabetes Association, South Texas Affiliate, Inc., P.O. Box 12946, Austin, TX 78711.)

Diabetes: Controlling It the Easy Way by Stanley Mirsky, M.D., and Joan Rattner Heilman. New York: Random House, 1982.

Diabetes: The Glucograf Method for Normalizing Blood Sugar by Richard K. Bernstein. New York: Crown Publishers, 1981.

How to Live with Diabetes by Henry Dolger, M.D., and Bernard Seeman. New York: W. W. Norton, 1977.

Joslin Diabetes Manual, ed. Leo J. Krall. Eleventh Edition, Philadelphia: Lea & Febiger, 1978.

Laurel's Kitchen (cookbook) by Carol Flinders, Godfrey Bronwen and Laurel Robertson. New York: Bantam Books, 1976.

The Baby Team by Donald R. Coustan, M.D., and Sheila Garvey, R.N. Monoject Division of Sherwood Medical, 1831 Olive Street, St. Louis, MO 63103 ($2.50, available by writing company).

The Diabetic's Book by June Biermann and Barbara Toohey. New York: J. P. Tarcher and Co., 1981.

The Diabetes Sports and Exercise Book by June Biermann and Barbara Toohey. Philadelphia: J. B. Lippincott and Company, 1977.

You Can't Catch Diabetes From a Friend (for children) by Lynne Kipnis and Susan Adler. Gainesville, Florida: Triad Scientific Publishers, 1979.

Every diabetic ought to have a copy of the *Physician's Desk Manual* or a similar work that tells you what medications are composed of and which ones might interact poorly with insulin or anything else you're taking for diabetes control. That way, if your physician recommends a drug for, say, your child's measles, you can check to see whether that drug might interact poorly with anything your child is taking for diabetes control.

IX. FREE EDUCATIONAL MATERIALS

Among other booklets available from the Juvenile Diabetes Foundation, you might write for:

What You Should Know About the Student with Diabetes
Having Children: A Guide for the Diabetic Woman
Parent to Parent: Your Baby Has Diabetes

Available from the Monoject Division of Sherwood Medical (1831 Olive St., St. Louis, MO 63103):

An Insulin Injection Site Locator—A wonderful chart, which comes with its own grease pencil for easy erasures to help you plan site changes. Also:
How to Take Insulin booklet

Booklets available from B-D (Becton, Dickinson & Co., Consumer Products, P.O. Box 5000, Rochelle Park, NJ 07662):

Site Selection and Rotation
Drawing and Injecting Insulin
Exercise and its Benefits

Dining Out Made Simple
Answers to Questions About Sick Days
Vacation Travel and Diabetes

Booklet available from Pfizer Laboratories (235 East 42nd St., New York, NY 10017):
Understanding Your Diabetes

Ames Company puts out a free newspaper called *Diabetes in the News.* If you wish to order it, write to: 233 East Erie Street, Suite 712, Chicago, IL 60611.

INDEX

of, 22–24, 36, 46, 54, 65–66
at parties, 66–67
primary physicians for, 5
reactions of, to diabetes, 87–88
remissions in, 14
"renal threshold" of, 16
responsibility for self fostered in, 84–85
in school, 66
selecting physicians for, 10–11
siblings of, 84
sleep and complications in, 52–54
snowflake cataracts in, 190
in solitary sports, 72, 109
teachers of, 61–63
traveling with, 74–80
vomiting, 14, 30–31
Children's Hospital, Philadelphia, Pa., 7
chloramphenicol, 137
cholesterol levels, 112, 210
chuckling, 133
Cidicol, 57
cigarette smoking, 107, 189
Clinilog, 20
Clinitest Two-Drop urine test, 18–19
Cohen, Walter, 130
cold remedies, 138–139
colleges, choice of, 104
color-blind people, reflectance colormeters and, 21–22
coma, diabetic, 4, 26–30, 34
  common causes of, 26–27
  symptoms of, 27–28
  treatment for, 5, 27–30
  unconsciousness unnecessary for, 27
Compazine, 30–31, 57
condoms, 147–148
constipation, 31, 194
contact lenses, 189
Continuous Ambulatory Peritoneal Disease (CAPD), 191
contraception, 146–148, 160
convulsions, 31–32, 35
Copenhagen, University Hospital of, 107
corticosteroids, 136
cortisone, 57, 198

costs, 85, 177
cough medicines, 57, 139
counseling:
  for family, 6
  for teens, 102, 109
Cousins, Norman, 133
crabs, 166
crankiness, 4, 24–25
creatinine clearance, 156
crying, anger vented by, 99
Cunningham, Barry, 119
cuts, 83

Daniel, C. W., 113
decongestants, 136
dehydration, in DKA, 28
deliveries, childbirth, 158
dental care, 129–131
  brushing teeth, 129
  flossing, 129
dentists, diabetes diagnosed by, 12
depression, 102
  in children, 85–87
  in teens, 102
dermopathy, diabetic, 198
dextrometers, 22n, 152
dextrose, 83
Dextrosol, 32–33
Dextrostix Reagent Strips, 21
diabetes, causes of, 103–104, 212–214
Diabetes Care, 22, 45, 50, 143
Diabetes Education Center, 109
diabetes pills, medications mixed with, 135–139
Diabetes: The Glucograf Method for Normalizing Blood Sugar (Bernstein), 19, 32, 111, 145, 195
diabetic keto-acidosis (DKA), *see* keto-acidosis, diabetic
Diabetic Retinopathy (L'Esperance and James), 190
Diabetic Retinopathy Study, 188
Diabetic's Book, The (Biermann and Toohey), 53
diabetologists, 10–11
  referrals for, 11
Dial-A-Dietician, 112
dialysis, 191